Instructor's Manual to Accompany

Critical Thinking in Nursing:
An Interactive Approach

M. GAIE RUBENFELD, RN, MS
Assistant Professor
Department of Nursing
Eastern Michigan University
Ypsilanti, Michigan

BARBARA K. SCHEFFER, RN, MS
Assistant Professor
Department of Nursing
Eastern Michigan University
Ypsilanti, Michigan

J.B. Lippincott Company
Philadelphia

Acquisitions Editor: Donna L. Hilton, RN, BSN
Ancillary Coordinator: Doris S. Wray
Coordinating Editorial Assistant: Susan M. Keneally
Compositor: Richard G. Hartley
Printer/Binder: R. R. Donnelly - Crawfordsville

Copyright © 1995, by J.B. Lippincott Company. All rights reserved. No part of this book may be used or reproduced in any manner whatsoever without written permission except for brief quotations embodied in critical articles and reviews. Printed in the United States of America. For information write J.B. Lippincott Company, 227 East Washington Square, Philadelphia, Pennsylvania 19106.

6 5 4 3 2 1

Library of Congress Cataloging-in-Publications Data
Rubenfeld, M. Gaie

    Instructor's manual to accompany critical thinking in nursing: an interactive approach / M. Gaie Rubenfeld, Barbara K. Scheffer.
        p.   cm.
    Includes bibliographical references and index.
    ISBN 0-397-55248-3

    1. Nursing-Philosophy. 2. Critical Thinking. 3. Nursing-Problems, exercises, etc. I. Scheffer, Barbara K. II. Title.
    [DNLM: 1. Nursing Process. 2. Thinking. WY 100 R895c 1995]
RT84.5R83 1995
610.73-dc20
DNLM/DLC
for Library of Congress   94-28466
                                                                                                 CIP

Any procedure or practice described in this book should be applied by the health-care practitioner under appropriate supervision in accordance with professional standards of care used with regard to the unique circumstances that apply in each practice situation. Care has been taken to confirm the accuracy of information presented and to describe generally accepted practices. However, the authors, editors, and publisher cannot accept any responsibility for errors or omissions or for any consequences from application of information in this book and make no warranty express or implied, with respect to the contents of this book.

Every effort has been made to ensure drug selections and dosages are in accordance with current recommendations and practice. Because of ongoing research, changes in government regulations and the constant flow of information on drug therapy, reactions and interactions, the reader is cautioned to check the package insert for each drug for indications, dosages, warnings, and precautions, particularly if the drug is new or infrequently used.

Table of Contents

Introduction 1

Chapter 1   Thinking..7

Chapter 2   Doing 13

Chapter 3   THINKING and DOING and the Nursing Process:
The HOW of Great Nursing 18

Chapter 4   Application of THINKING and DOING in the Nursing Process..23

Chapter 5   Nursing Conclusions 27

Chapter 6   Major Nursing Conclusions of Assessment 32

Chapter 7   Health Detectives: Data Collection and Data Analysis 37

Chapter 8   Making More Sense of Clues: Cluster Analysis 44

Chapter 9   Designing, Doing and Determining Quality of Care: a.k.a.
Planning, Implementing, and Evaluated 50

Chapter 10   Written and Verbal Communication
of Thinking and Doing..57

Chapter 11   Consequences of Thinking and Not
Thinking When Documenting 61

Chapter 12   Assessing a Complete Patient Situation..................................65

Chapter 13   Designing, Doing, and Determining Quality of Care
for Actual Problems with Multiple Related Factors...............70

Chapter 14   Designing, Doing, and Determining Quality of Care
for High-Risk Problems...74

Chapter 15   Designing, Doing, and Determining Quality of Care
for Wellness Issues, Interdisciplinary Problems,
and Problems for Referral..77

Chapter 16   Thinking into the Future: From Linear Equation
to Paradigm of Great Nursing..81

Introduction

This manual was designed to expand on the rationale behind the content and activities in the text, *Critical Thinking in Nursing: An Interactive Approach* and to suggest some teaching strategies. This introduction addresses general issues such as ways the book can be used in a variety of classroom and non-classroom settings, the underlying teaching strategies, unique classroom activities, incorporation of clinical activities, and methods for evaluating and grading student thinking and outcomes.

The remaining sections of this manual are arranged to correspond with the book chapters. Each section lists the key concepts and teaching objectives of the chapters, provides rationales and teaching options for each Action Learning exercise, and elaborates on the Thinking Log. In line with our strong beliefs about and values of relativistic thinking, we hope you will take these ideas as suggestions, not as the "right" approaches, and use the book in creative ways.

▶ Classroom and Non-classroom Settings for Use of the Text

The text can be used as a required text outside or within classroom situations. The text includes many independent activities and promotes extensive peer collaboration outside the classroom. An instructor could facilitate small study groups working through the chapters independently and use the clinical and classroom settings for clarification, testing, and applying the concepts.

If the book is used in a course primarily taught in the classroom, the methods used to reinforce the content may vary according to class size. The large lecture format continues to be a reality in all areas of teaching. Students in large groups can be placed into smaller groups of eight to ten within the large room. Each group can be given the same discussion or problem-solving task and the instructor can circulate around the room to provide guidance and input as the groups are working. After a set period of time, the groups can reconvene as the whole and each group may share (through their representative) the results of their thinking.

As a guideline, we have found the most cost-effective, ideal size for teaching critical thinking content to be a group of 20 to 22 students. Even this size group can be broken into smaller groups for many of the activities, but the sharing among 20 students takes much less time than it would with a larger group.

▶ Basic Strategies Used throughout the Text

We have found over many years of teaching and learning from nursing students that the strategies discussed below produce the best thinkers. (These strategies are also well supported by the educational research focused on learning and thinking skills.)

▷ Building on existing knowledge and thinking skills.

Students are not blank slates. They come with a whole repertoire of life experience and thinking skills for everyday living. By acknowledging these facts and identifying and enhancing what they already have, students can more quickly develop quality thinking in nursing.

▷ Multisensory learning methods.

Educational research has shown that skill and knowledge become integrated more quickly if students incorporate all their senses in the learning process—hearing, seeing, doing, feeling, touching, writing, drawing, describing, smelling. Extensive use of examples from everyday life as well as nursing also helps students make the connections necessary for retention.

▷ Relativistic approach.

An ongoing challenge for instructors is to help students tolerate ambiguity and recognize that no one "right" answer is necessarily appropriate in all situations. We have found the following strategies to be useful. Avoid linear, step-by-step formats; ask questions that require analysis rather than simple recall; stress the process of thinking as well as the *outcomes* of thinking; provide examples with a "good," "better," and "best" response; and verbalize the thinking processes you, as the instructor, use.

▷ **Reflection (knowing how you think).**

This has also been called metacognition. It is helpful to demonstrate this and use the "thinking" vocabulary identified in Chapter 1 in the text. The Thinking Log (diary) is useful in nurturing reflection, which is a new concept to many students. Students discover a whole new aspect to their being as they become reflective thinkers.

▷ **Role modeling thinking.**

Role modeling has long beenconsidered a valuable teaching method. Role modeling thinking is more challenging. First, thinking is abstract and not tangible. Second, to show it requires extra effort on the part of the instructor who, as an expert, has finely tuned, almost subconscious, thinking skills. Tracking back and slowing down your thinking to describe it to a beginner takes extra thought. We have found it easiest to practice with another instructor first.

▷ **Rewards.**

The concept of rewarding success is age-old. We found several low-cost techniques for rewarding the thinking processes as much as the outcomes of thinking. Extra credit points on quizzes, pencils, or hard candy as rewards for early classroom participation and compliments on verbalizing thinking have been effective. Students are also strongly encouraged to identify internal reward systems.

▷ **Humor.**

Humor is a wonderful elixir for anxiety. An open, friendly, sharing classroom atmosphere helps most students relax. Use of humorous illustrations, cartoons, or funny examples helps diminish anxiety and increase retention. Sharing funny examples of mistakes instructors have made in their own learning is especially helpful. The illustrations in the text are humorous examples of complex content.

▷ **Repetition.**

Retention of information, internalization, and application of learning occur more quickly when information is repeated. Repetition of basic information in increasingly complex situations is particularly helpful. The text is designed to continually use and develop skills learned in early chapters.

▷ **Collaboration.**

Collaboration has been the underlying themein education for the last decade. Although it is espoused in health care, students don't always see effective examples nor are they provided with useful opportunities to collaborate. We have stressed the need for peer collaboration as a way of nurturing a lifelong behavior that will promote the best nursing care. Students are instructed to seek classmate input, critiques, and suggestions with most of the Action Learning exercises. Collaboration is also incorporated in most of the classroom activities. Guidance is provided on how to use collaboration to the advantage of both student and patient.

▷ **Appreciation of feelings, values, and beliefs.**

The affective component of learning is valued for its impact on thinking. The degree of the impact varies depending on the student. Action Learning exercises are specifically designed to help students identify their values and beliefs and the impact of those values and beliefs on nursing conclusions and care.

▷ **Memory aids.**

The volume of information in nursing that needs to be committed to memory can be overwhelming. Many students profit from a discussion of how to find patterns or use mnemonic devices as memory aids. Memory is also enhanced by using analogies and real life examples. Having students design or diagram a concept in a personal interpretation helps them develop a sense of ownership of learning and also enhances retention of concepts.

▷ **Blending content knowledge and thinking.**

Content knowledge is limited for the beginning student, but most have some basic understanding of stress responses, nutrition, exercise, sleep, and elimination. As the students' content knowledge increases while they are concurrently taking other nursing courses, the complexity of nursing data and care can also increase. Case studies used in the book start with simple situations and then increase in complexity to allow for this growth in content knowledge. Students are also guided to use standardized plans as "triggers" to thinking so care can be individualized to a patient's unique needs.

▷ **Focusing on the "big picture."**

Many students learn best if they can see the "big picture" and get a clear sense of what they are aiming for. The nursing process is taught as a whole so that students appreciate what data are most important to collect, how planning is affected by data collection, how evaluation is affected by planning, and so forth. Once the whole is explored and appreciated, the details make more sense.

▶ **Selected Classroom Activities**

A variety of activities can be effective in the classroom to promote participation by all students and focus on the thinking modes. Setting the tone and expectations early in the course is helpful. We have asked students to use name cards with their first name printed in large dark letters. These cards can either be taped on them or their desks.

Name cards allow instructors to call on all students, not just those who spontaneously participate, at some point during each class. The major advantages of this technique are that the instructor becomes familiar with all the students by name, and more importantly, all students recognize that they will have an opportunity, at least once during each class, to share their thinking. This technique, although increasing interaction, also produces anxiety for some students. How the student response is handled can diminish anxiety. For example, no matter what the response the student can be praised for trying with comments such as, "That's close," or "Good start; who would like to add to that?" or if the student is really "off," consider saying, "Let me rephrase the question so you can think about it a different way."

A second technique that can encourage peer critique and collaboration is related to care planning. Students are asked to write their care plans on large sheets of paper or opened grocery bags. The plans are taped on the walls around the classroom and small groups of students are assigned to critique each plan. Guidelines for critiquing are provided in the *Tracking Nursing Thinking Checklist* in Appendix B.

To assist students with early data collection before they have a clinical experience, a videotaped interview is helpful. We videotaped an instructor doing a health assessment of another instructor and one with a volunteer "patient." Students viewed the tape either outside of class or during class and had to identify relevant data, their hunches and supporting data, and their major conclusions of assessment.

Once students have a corresponding clinical assignment, data from their clinical patients can be used for the classroom activities. When working in groups, the group selects data from one of the member's clinical patients as the focus for the activity assigned at that time.

One of our most creative activities was used at the end of a course. The purpose was to provide a memorable summary and review as well as to allow students to personally create and teach. Educational research supports that teaching something is the best way to learn. Students were randomly assigned to groups of four or five. Each group was assigned to review three book chapters and develop a 10-minute presentation of their assigned content. Students were encouraged to be as creative as possible in ways that would always be remembered to convey the key concepts of their chapters. The student presentations included the use of crossword puzzles; game shows; and skits with unique props, music, and costumes. They were funny and greatly enhanced learning.

▶ Evaluating and Grading

Methods for evaluating and grading were developed that nurture and focus on the *process* of thinking as well as on the *outcomes* of thinking. Students earn classroom points for sharing their ideas and thoughts with the group.

Quizzes may be used to evaluate the content learned in the text and course. One form of quiz-making and quiz-taking was particularly helpful and less anxiety producing. Each student was instructed to develop and submit two questions related to the content that had been presented to date. The instructor reviewed all the questions and selected ten for the quiz. The ten questions were typed and distributed to all students in advance with the understanding that three questions would be chosen by the instructor for the actual quiz given in class. Students were also involved in grading the questions by exchanging quizzes as specific parts of the answer were discussed. In most cases, several answers were read and students decided which one was best. The instructor reviewed any answers that needed more attention.

Students can also be evaluated on their care plans. Some care plans are developed from data provided in class and some from data about the student's clinical patient. The TNT Checklist can be used to guide the development of the care plan as well as the self-evaluation and instructor evaluation of the care plan. This checklist is discussed throughout the latter chapters of the text and is also provided in Appendix B.

▶ Additional Resources

Every day new resources that focus on critical thinking are becoming available in nursing. The field of education has had rich sources of information for quite some time. A brief bibliography specifically helpful for teaching critical thinking and nursing process are listed at the end of the book. Many of the references address teaching methods as well as the research and content on thinking. Instructors are encouraged to use this as a beginning. Regular computer searches using *critical thinking* as one of the descriptive search labels will yield further information.

1

Thinking

This chapter sets the tone for the book by providing a method to explore the various types of thinking used by nurses. It focuses heavily on self-exploration of thinkers and contains eight Action Learning exercises and the first Thinking Log.

In this chapter, teaching strategies that reinforce thinking are essential to developing students' attitudes for the remaining parts of the book. This book is somewhat different from most texts in that it focuses on the process of thinking as well as on the outcomes of thinking. This may produce some initial anxiety for students as they wonder how they will be evaluated. Because anxiety is counterproductive to higher order thinking, every attempt should be made to decrease the typical anxiety that occurs when new ideas and concepts are being learned.

Consistent, positive reinforcement when the student uses thinking processes and interactions with peers should allay some of the anxiety and help students begin to value those processes. Clear explanations of the focus on the thinking processes as well as on the outcomes of thinking are helpful, as is role modeling of thinking by the instructor.

▶ **Key Content Areas**

Classification of Thinking Modes
Exploration of Personal Thinking Style

8 ▼ Thinking

▶ Teaching Objectives

- Help students differentiate the five modes of thinking.
- Provide a nonthreatening atmosphere for students' self-exploration of thinking styles.
- Set a low anxiety-producing learning atmosphere for this and future chapters.

Rationale and Teaching Options for Action Learning Exercises

▷▷▷▷▷▷Action Learning #1: Draw Your Thinking Cap

▷ **Rationale**: Many reasons for this activity are listed in the discussion section following the exercise. In addition, there is an immediate message to readers that this book is active and interactive.

▷ **Teaching Options**: The "thinking cap" can be a personal symbol for each student. Some students actually have caps they wear when they study. Discussions of thinking caps can lead to a sharing of other thinking aids. Some students wear a favorite shirt, bathrobe, or pants to study, for example.

Discussions of these personal thinking aids can be light and humorous. A non—self-conscious faculty member might even venture into the classroom wearing his or her favorite thinking outfit — the one worn while reading, writing, or thinking at home.

For the student who says that he or she cannot draw anything, having an opportunity to see other students' caps can start the ball rolling. At the risk of stating the obvious, we recommend decreasing student anxiety by not forcing anyone to share this early drawing. In our experience, many students freely share their hats, so that lively discussion occurs. These hats can become elaborate, with flaps, antennae, feathers, straps, brims, and many other symbolic parts.

▷▷▷▷▷▷Action Learning #2: Can You Remember?

▷ **Rationale**: Information recall may seem to be a simple mode of thinking. However, many individualized approaches are used. Because nursing has so many facts to be remembered, beginning students sometimes feel overwhelmed. Having students think about their memory abilities allows them to actively address what may otherwise be taken for granted and increase opportunities for enhancing existing skills.

An important part of this learning exercise is the acknowledgement that everything doesn't have to be memorized—that it's OK to look things up. Some students need initial guidance in learning how to look things up. A discussion of study habits often occurs when students share perceptions of total recall thinking. Sharing and collaboration provide ideas for enhancing existing skills.

▷ **Teaching Options:** Group discussion works well. The questions posed in the discussion section following the exercise can be used as starters. If there is insufficient time for a full group discussion, students can be encouraged to share their ideas in small groups or an assignment can be made for students to find and talk with someone who uses a memory aid different from theirs.

▷▷▷▷▷▷Action Learning #3: Personal Habits

▷ **Rationale**: Helping students relate this thinking mode (HABITS) to their existing life experience helps them recognize they don't have to develop totally new skills, they just need to add to existing ones.

▷ **Teaching Options:** In addition to class discussion of habit thinking, students who are in clinical settings could be asked to list thinking habits that they see nurses use. Discussion of such findings could focus on the positive and negative aspects of those habits.

▷▷▷▷▷▷Action Learning #4: Inquiry into Bertha's Body

▷ **Rationale:** This exercise situation is purposefully "tricky," so that students can see the complexities of inquiry thinking. Because premature conclusions are the antithesis of inquiry and because biases are not always immediately obvious to beginning students, this exercise focuses on those pitfalls. The more sophisticated possible conclusions, as most experienced nurses will confirm, are that Bertha could be pregnant or have a tumor, ascites, or renal failure.

Discussions of inquiry thinking are good opportunities to explore students' attitudes toward authorities—be they persons or written works. Useful questions might be, "Are authorities always right?" or "Who qualifies as an authority?"

▷ **Teaching Options:** Other clinical examples would be helpful to illustrate inquiry thinking. Students could share patient situations with each other to see how many possible conclusions could be made.

A nursing research report could be used to stimulate inquiry thinking. A classic approach to research critique could be used or adapted to the abilities of beginning students.

Other nonnursing examples could be used to provide students with inquiry practice. Students could watch a movie, read a story, read or watch a news report, or observe a human interaction and do a critical analysis. If controversial subjects are chosen, students have the added benefit of values and ethics clarification. Formal debate is the classic arena for inquiry-style thinking.

▷▷▷▷▷Action Learning #5: New Ideas and Creativity

▷ **Rationale**: Because creativity is key to individualized nursing care, it is important for students to gain an appreciation of this form of thinking early in their careers. Beginning students have had limited opportunity to try creative nursing approaches, so they may find it easier to cite nonnursing examples of their creativity. Seeing the creativity of their peers allows them to see other students as individuals as well as using those ideas to "trigger" their own creativity.

▷ **Teaching Options:** This is one of our particular favorite modes of thinking. With a little extra effort, students can be encouraged to have a creativity show—to bring in examples of their creative work and share them with others. Students could put on a talent show or a cooking show-off or have an art exhibit, for example. Such an activity could be coordinated with activities of other student groups such as the Student Nurses' Association and used as a fund-raiser, or just be a happening. Nurturing creativity is a laudable trait in nursing faculty.

For enlightened discussions and suggestions for nurturing creativity, Cameron's book listed in the bibliography of *Critical Thinking in Nursing: An Interactive Approach* is an excellent source.

▷▷▷▷▷Action Learning #6: How You Think

▷ **Rationale**: The rationale for this activity is probably self-evident for a book focused on thinking. In many later exercises, students are asked to relate to their own ways of thinking, so this sets the stage. It is often not until someone is specifically asked to describe how he or she thinks that it becomes clear how difficult this can be. Even if students have only general comments at first, this exercise can be an impetus for rich discussions.

Thinking ▼ 11

▷ **Teaching Options:** Instructor role modeling may be helpful; giving a description of how you think shows students how to start. Sometimes students can describe how they believe someone else thinks more easily than they can describe their own approaches. Allowing students to describe the thinking of a character in a movie or book or a person well known to them can give them practice with descriptions. Caution is needed here to avoid jumping to unvalidated conclusions. It is helpful to encourage students to be descriptive when supporting their beliefs about how "someone else is thinking." This can be done by asking, "What data support your conclusions?" After such practice, they may be able to describe their own thinking more easily.

▷▷▷▷▷▷Action Learning #7: Metacognition Check

▷ **Rationale**: The language used to describe thinking is sometimes unfamiliar. Practice with the thinking vocabulary will allow students to become familiar with ways to describe their thinking.

▷ **Teaching Options:** These vocabulary words could be incorporated into written and verbal reports in other nursing courses. Students could be given extra credit for using these and other such descriptors in class. A brief paper describing their thinking about their thinking could also provide extra credit.

▷▷▷▷▷▷Action Learning #8: What Makes Your Thinking Unique?

▷ **Rationale**: To fully understand how one thinks, it is vital to appreciate one's uniqueness. The factors that make thinking unique are described in the paragraphs preceding this exercise. Having students study each factor and relate it to a thinking issue both increases their self-awareness and provides a review of the preceding content.

▷ **Teaching Options:** This exercise could be done in many ways. Early in a course, students could be asked to introduce and describe themselves according to the seven factors. Or, if they know each other well, their descriptions could be written on cards. Other students could then try to match the cards with the person.

Thinking Log #1

This first Thinking Log is designed to help students review what they have learned and relate it to the learning outcomes at the beginning of the chapter. This activity encourages students to adapt this method of review into their study habits. It promotes thinking by helping students see connections between content and learning outcomes and focuses on multisensory learning with the use of writing to express thoughts. Education research supports the strong connections between writing clearly and thinking clearly. The thinking logs in general are designed as journals. "Journaling" as it is being used in other areas of education provides concrete evidence of thinking and reasoning, a skill of great value in nursing.

The format for each Thinking Log varies throughout the book. Even though later logs do not ask students to review the learning outcomes of those chapters, students, ideally, will do such a review for each chapter or could be encouraged to do so as an assignment.

2

Doing

Chapter 2 is also essential to setting the tone for the learning associated with this book. All nursing programs teach beginning students many tasks such as bed making, vital signs assessment, transfer techniques, or medication administration. If those tasks are taught without a concurrent focus on thinking, the students run the risk of developing only habitual nursing approaches. Equally unproductive is teaching students about thinking without combining it with the teaching related to psychomotor skills. Both of these approaches result in students being unable to integrate thinking and doing.

This chapter discusses what nurses do in terms that the beginning student can understand. At the same time, some of the complexities of what nurses do are presented to show why doing cannot occur without thinking.

▶ Key Content Areas

Listing and Discussing What Nurses Do
Exploring Factors That Affect Doing
Interrelating Thinking and Doing

▶ Teaching Objectives

- Help students explore their present knowledge about what nurses do.
- Simplify the doing aspects of nursing enough so that beginners can understand the various tasks without losing sight of their complexity.

- Use nonjudgmental approaches while helping students examine their values, beliefs, and expectations about nursing.
- Acknowledge the usual thinking approaches used by beginners while, at the same time, instilling an appreciation of aiming for higher level relativistic thinking.

Rationale and Teaching Options for Action Learning Exercises

Action Learning #9: What DO Nurses DO?

▷ **Rationale:** This is an example of a recurrent theme in this book—helping students identify their present knowledge about some aspect of nursing so that new information can be added to what already exists. Most students come to nursing with some knowledge about what nurses do. Some of those ideas are realistic; some are less so. Some students have worked in health care delivery and may have lots of information, whereas others have only media portrayals of nursing as their knowledge base. Having students share their lists with each other can be beneficial to those who have no health care experience. It can also help students who have extensive knowledge to organize and clarify their information.

▷ **Teaching Options:** This list could be created as an in-class discussion with students brainstorming while someone records the list on a blackboard or large paper. Students who are concurrently in clinical situations could be asked to make their lists as they observe nurses at work. However, if the latter approach is taken, there is a risk of some students never listing their pre-nursing conceptions. If those observations of what nurses do are stereotypical of media portrayals, for example, the student has not had an opportunity to discuss the reality or nonreality of those perceptions. Such exploration can provide for rich discussion and could be done during a pre- or postconference.

Students could also be asked to watch a TV show or movie or read a book about nurses and, from those, list what nurses do. Such an assignment would allow for a valuable exploration of nursing's image and the reality of that image.

Another alternative would be to take the DOING List presented in this chapter and ask students to look for examples, either in the real world or in the media, of nurses doing those things. The advantage to this approach is that it would reinforce the learning of the list. The disadvantage is similar to that mentioned in the first part of this discussion—students would have less opportunity to explore their existing perceptions.

Doing ▼ 15

Instructors may want to review the Thinking Log at the end of this chapter before deciding on a teaching strategy. This log asks students to explore doing by talking to an experienced nurse.

▷▷▷▷▷▷Action Learning #10: Effect of Values, Beliefs, and Expectations on Nursing Care

▷ **Rationale:** The importance of having students honestly explore their values, beliefs, and expectations cannot be stressed enough. Without such self-exploration, students may believe they can segment their minds and think and act in nursing in an objective manner. As any experienced nurse knows, such objectivity is unrealistic and nonhuman. Students can mistakenly get the message that they must be "better" than others and stifle their feelings. This can lead to robot-like nursing where patients rarely see nurses as human beings. Open exploration, where anything can be safely acknowledged, is the first step in students' learning about how they can work with their values, beliefs, and expectations, change them if necessary, and balance them with caring approaches in nursing.

A second and equally important aspect of this exercise is that both patients have the same nursing diagnosis. Having two value-laden patient situations with identical face-value nursing implications allows students to see how the "doing," while seemingly similar, could be very different as a result of the nurse's values and beliefs, not the individual differences of the patients.

▷ **Teaching Options:** Ideally, students will be learning or will have had classes on values clarification or ethics about the time they are doing this exercise. If such is the case, instructors could bring in that content to reinforce the learning. Obviously, this one exercise is merely an appetite whetter for learning about values, beliefs, and expectations.

Most experienced instructors could easily devise many situations similar to Dolly's and Monty's. Students concurrently in clinical settings could identify patient situations in which their values, beliefs, and expectations affected or potentially affected what they did for those patients.

The value of discussing "real" patients is that students can explore what they really did rather than what they think they would have done. Ideally, students could complete this workbook exercise *and* analyze one of their own patient care situations so they could compare what they think they would have done with what they actually did. This would add a rich layer of reality to this self-exploration.

It is critical in exercises such as this one that instructors maintain a nonjudgmental tone during student discussions. If students get the message that they "shouldn't" have a certain value, for example, they will not openly explore those values. Nurturing INQUIRY thinking is effective in helping students examine the basis for their beliefs, values, and expectations. Not until they recognize the difference between values/beliefs and facts can they choose which values/beliefs they want to keep and which they want to modify.

▷▷▷▷▷▷Action Learning #11: Moving Beyond a Beginner's Way of Gaining Knowledge

▷ **Rationale:** The intent in this exercise is to help students learn how to incorporate content knowledge with clinical practice. As most instructors will recognize, this is an ongoing challenge to teaching in nursing. Students who can read books and repeat that information back on an objective test do not automatically apply the thinking needed to adapt that information in a patient situation.

This exercise uses diet counseling as an example because most beginning students know something about diets already, even if they have not had nursing courses related to such content. This exercise allows for building on students' present knowledge.

Dietary intervention was also chosen because several different approaches can be found in textbooks and articles. Through their sharing, students can appreciate that many approaches can be used and using only one source of information is not the best way to understand the complexities of nursing interventions.

▷ **Teaching Options:** For instructors using this workbook with more advanced students, a more complex example could be used that shows students how to gain knowledge and then apply it in a nursing situation. However, when using other examples, it is helpful to select ones where the knowledge base in nursing is not "cut and dried." Because there are many different approaches to nursing interventions for weight reduction, students can find a variety of approaches in the literature. This reinforces the message that multiple sources should be used for optimal learning and optimal application of that learning.

Other areas of nursing where the literature presents many different approaches to consider are, among others, skin care, grief counseling, intermittent urinary catheterization, tracheostomy care, infant feeding schedules, and stress management. Using a controversial area of care will enrich this learning exercise.

Doing 17

▷▷▷▷▷ Action Learning #12: What Is the Nurse DOING and What Factors Are Affecting the DOING?

▷ **Rationale:** This exercise allows students to integrate the knowledge gained in this chapter. A nurse working with a patient being discharged from the hospital is used as an example so that a wide range of nursing activities can be seen.

▷ **Teaching Options:** Any nursing situation more relevant to students' current area of practice could be used instead of this one. Students may also be able to identify additional examples of "doing" from a personally relevant situation. Instructors may be able to reinforce other concurrent learning by using an alternative situation.

Regardless of the situation used in this exercise, the discussion aspect probably needs to be maintained. By comparing approaches with their classmates, students can see that there are many acceptable approaches and many ways to think about factors affecting the doing. Such discussions can reinforce relativistic thinking especially if the students are reminded that they are starting to use relativistic thinking effectively.

Thinking Log #2

In keeping with the DOING focus, this log asks students to do something in addition to recording their thinking. Students who are concurrently in a clinical situation will find it easy to interview a nurse. Those who are not in a clinical setting may need assistance in finding a nurse to interview. Other nursing faculty members may be considered as interview candidates if getting students to agencies is a problem.

One of the most important aspects of this exercise is the fourth question they will pose to the nurse—"How much of your day is spent thinking?" This question may surprise some nurses, delight others, and possibly stymie a few. The students are likely to get many different responses; the sharing component of this exercise should be emphasized so that the group can benefit from all of the answers.

Copyright © 1995 J. B. Lippincott Co., Instructor's Manual to Accompany Critical Thinking in Nursing: An Interactive Approach

3

THINKING and DOING and the Nursing Process: The HOW of Great Nursing

The focus of this chapter is a nontraditional approach to the nursing process. The overall picture of the process is examined in a situational context before the details of the components of the nursing process are explored in later chapters.

No specific theoretical framework for nursing is advocated in this chapter, or for that matter, in the entire book. However, an overview of significant theoretical content is provided. Faculty will want to translate the content presented in the text to the theoretical orientation used in their curricula. The content of this chapter, and the whole book, will easily fit with any theoretical framework.

The nursing process is described as the four phases of assessing, planning, implementing, and evaluating after the original nursing process work done by Yura and Walsh. A note is made of the commonly used five-phase process with nursing diagnosis as its own phase. In the authors' view (and this is stated in the text), diagnosing is part of assessing and therefore is not considered as a separate fifth phase. If the five-step process is preferred, a brief explanation of this difference between the book and the students' curriculum might allay any confusion.

THINKING and DOING ▼ 19

▶ Key Content Areas

The Nursing Process and How It Fits into a Formula for Great Nursing
Historical Context of the Nursing Process
The Components of the Nursing Process and Their Possible Sequences
Thinking and Doing Parts of the Components of the Nursing Process

▶ Teaching Objectives

- Promote an appreciation of the nursing process within a context of great nursing.
- Help students value the patient, content knowledge, thinking, and themselves as essential components of great nursing.
- Help students understand what the nursing process is and how thinking and doing are part of that process.
- Promote an understanding of the process as more than four separate components.
- Contrast standard recipes with individualized care.

Rationale and Teaching Options for Action Learning Exercises

Action Learning #13: _____'s Definition of Great Nursing

▷ **Rationale:** This exercise in self-reflection provides a personal ownership of an ideal early in students' careers. It becomes their definition of great nursing by which they can monitor their growth as nurses.

▷ **Teaching Options:** Other means to stimulate students to develop a personal definition of nursing would be to ask them to list the characteristics of "poor" nursing and then look for opposite characteristics. Sometimes students can use "horror stories" about less than optimal care to do this exercise.

It may also be helpful to have students do a composite definition in class, display the final product in the classroom, and periodically return to it for review. Yet another helpful exercise is to have students define nursing from a patient's perspective, a nurse's perspective, and a health care executive's perspective. They could then discuss how these might be different.

Students concurrently in a clinical setting could list examples of great nursing that they have seen or experienced in their work.

Action Learning #14: Find the Nursing Care WITH Mr. Steinberg

▷ **Rationale:** Helping students see the importance of doing nursing care *with*, rather than *to*, patients cannot be reinforced too much. Many health care systems, especially inpatient settings, often ignore the fact that patients have the right to make decisions about their own health. Students see many examples of the power over patient's health being usurped by health care providers. When that occurs a vital part of the nursing process (patient participation) is missing and the thought processes so important to great nursing are stifled.

▷ **Teaching Options:** This exercise leads well into discussions of empowerment, power, and patient rights. If content on ethics from other courses can be integrated into this exercise, the discussion will be strengthened.

An actual patient case, rather than this written one, could be used for this exercise. Students could analyze a situation they were involved in and determine when they did things to a patient rather than with the patient.

Another similar learning experience could be achieved by having students pretend to be a patient in role playing. One student could do things to the patient, after which the feelings of the patient could be discussed.

This exericise could be combined with a laboratory experience in which students learn to do hygiene care. One student could brush another's teeth, wash the face, and comb the hair. The student could do it first as a "to-the-patient" procedure and then change the approach so that it is done with the patient directing the tasks. Students who were the recipients of care could then list how differently they felt in each situation.

Action Learning #15: Where to Start

▷ **Rationale:** Many texts show or imply that the nursing process is a linear set of steps moving from assessing to planning to implementing to evaluating, in that order. There is a concerted effort in this text to avoid any implication of a linear process. Linearity says to students—here's a recipe; just follow it. A recipe message does little to stimulate thinking and is not grounded in the reality of nursing practice where almost nothing occurs in a linear fashion.

This activity focuses, again, on helping students identify what thinking comes naturally to their minds, building on their present thinking styles.

▷ **Teaching Options:** Many examples could be used from the instructor's repertoire of practice situations or from those the students have in their experience. Any situation could be used to illustrate the nonlinear process.

If students have limited clinical experience, a nonnursing example would work well to illustrate the content here. Sequences of activities from everyday situations might relate to cooking, preparing for a party, repairing a car, putting together a jigsaw puzzle, and so on. Ask students to explain what they did first, what they thought about first, and why they thought that way. Such an analysis will allow students to see how different people approach the same task in different but equally effective ways.

It is important to acknowledge the thinking patterns of students who tend to be rigid and naturally linear and to equally acknowledge the thinking of students who are seemingly disorganized. Neither group of students should get the message that their approaches are wrong. Rather, they could be gently helped to explore new ways to enhance existing styles. Both groups of students may need guidance and nurturing to analyze their thinking and determine why they are more rigid or why they are more disorganized. Again, recognizing what currently exists is a preliminary step to growth and change.

▷▷▷▷▷▷Action Learning #16: Identifying Components as the Nursing Process Is Used

▷ **Rationale:** This activity allows students to see a "big picture" of the nursing process. The case is long so that the interrelationships and lack of a linear sequence can be seen. The situation is fairly simple in terms of its subject matter; many novice students have had some experience with a child who is a finicky eater. At the same time, the situation is complex and realistic in terms of what a student nurse must think about and do.

▷ **Teaching Options:** This exercise could be done in class with the instructor going through the case paragraph by paragraph, asking students to identify the nursing process component. Done as a class activity, there may be rich discussions of areas that are not necessarily straightforward. For example, where does planning end and implementing begin? How much implementation is being done at the same time the nurse assesses the situation? Class discussion also provides opportunities to explore students' biases and preconceived ideas about how to get Jesse to eat better and how to teach parenting skills.

Another option for this exercise is to use a movie or videotape of a nurse at work and have the students look for the components of the nursing process. Unfortunately, popular movies rarely depict nurses in realistic situations.

22 ▼ THINKING and DOING

Most movies with nurses could serve as negative examples from which students could identify what nurses could and should be doing in them.

▷▷▷▷▷ Action Learning #17: Thinking and the Nursing Process

▷ **Rationale:** This exercise is a companion exercise to #16. The two parts of the activity, identifying the components of the process and identifying the thinking modes, are separated on purpose so students can concentrate on one and then the other. This activity provides a review of the THINK mnemonic from Chapter 1. This repetition increases retention.

▷ **Teaching Options:** The same options presented in the previous activity are applicable to this activity. Note that the answers to #16 and #17 are provided in the summary following #17. If possible, encourage students to wait to read this section until they have tried their hands at the two exercises.

Thinking Log #3

This Thinking Log encourages students to consider things beyond what they have read in the text. It was designed to promote an attitude that books, even great ones (such as this one—Ahem!), can never include all possible answers. Writing their thoughts promotes organization of thinking. Sharing thoughts with classmates continues to organize thinking, nurture peer collaboration, enhance feedback, and encourage modification to achieve even better ideas.

4

Application of THINKING and DOING in the Nursing Process

Chapter 4 continues to focus on thinking about the whole of the nursing process with more examples. This continued focus provides the repetition needed to begin to internalize the major concepts of the nursing process. Students are encouraged to grasp the "big picture" as clearly as possible so that the details in the next chapters will make more sense.

The chapter also provides an opportunity to demonstrate existing thinking skills and addresses the issue of self-concept in relation to thinking skills. It encourages students to gain insight into how they think, how they feel about their thinking skills, and how they feel about comparing their thinking with that of their classmates.

The third major focus of this chapter is to track the thinking that occurs while using the nursing process. This abstract process (thinking) is illustrated through a specific case where Ken, a student nurse, uses his thinking skills. Ken can be viewed as a peer to whom students can relate as they learn.

Application of THINKING and DOING

▶ Key Content Areas

Examining the Students' Ability to Think through a Simple Nursing Situation and Identify Feelings about Their Personal Thinking Skills

Tracking Thinking through the Whole Nursing Process

▶ Teaching Objectives

- Identify, apply, and nurture existing thinking skills.
- Provide a nonthreatening atmosphere for examining feelings about personal thinking skills and peer collaboration.
- Analyze the thinking used by the student nurse when he applied the complete nursing process to provide care in a simple nursing situation.

Rationale and Teaching Options for Action Learning Exercises

▷▷▷▷▷▷Action Learning #18: The Big Think

▷ **Rationale:** This activity is designed to allow the student to achieve several outcomes. The first is to practice using and identifying existing personal thinking approaches with a simple nursing situation. The second is to examine differences from and similarities with peers' thinking. The third is to acknowledge feelings about personal thinking approaches both separately and as compared to peers.

▷ **Teaching Options:** The 12 questions to be answered in relation to this exercise can also be done independently outside of class, in small groups, or in a large lecture. If used in a classroom setting, it is best to instruct all students to develop their own responses and then have the instructor randomly select students to share their responses as opposed to just calling on the students who raise their hands.

The questions are designed to focus on the INQUIRY and KNOWING HOW YOU THINK modes as the student is asked to explain why each question was answered as it was. It will be helpful to nurture and encourage students to describe their thinking in as much detail as possible as opposed to allowing them to simply say, "it just makes sense to do it this way." It may be helpful to ask the student to elaborate on why it makes sense to reinforce the process of thinking as well as the outcome of thinking.

Guidance can be provided on how to share information with peers and how to deal with feelings while sharing. It will be helpful to reinforce the value of comparing different approaches. It may also be helpful for instructors to describe their thinking styles. This modeling can decrease the anxiety that frequently occurs when students begin to focus on their thinking styles and personal thinking approaches used for developing the answers. Acknowledgement of the possibility of several effective responses to each question as opposed to there being a "right" answer is important to nurturing relativistic thinking.

Action Learning #19: Developing a Goal and Objectives

▷ **Rationale:** This activity allows the student to deduce what would be effective format language for patient goals and objectives by examining the sample care plan provided in this chapter. It also can nudge students to seek out useful sources of information necessary to design nursing care when their content knowledge is limited. The discussion section for #19 includes one effective way of developing a goal and objective.

▷ **Teaching Options:** The instructor can assist the students in analyzing the format and function of the goal and objectives in the sample care plan. For example, the instructor can ask questions such as, "What are the key elements in the goal statement?" (client centered, time frame, flow from nursing diagnosis). "What do you think is the purpose of the goal statement?" "How does the goal statement fit with the nursing diagnosis?" The same process of analysis can be done for objectives.

Alternative formats for goal statements and objectives can be introduced to fit with each nursing program's system of developing written plans of care.

If this activity is to be done outside of class, students could be required to write out a list of useful and current literature sources as well as identify persons who could provide information. If this activity is done in class, students could be divided into small groups with each group having a different textbook or article to read that would relate to Self-Care Deficit. The group would be required to find the relevant information and report back to the whole group with a citation for each reference. A discussion could follow focused on how to adjust the information gleaned from the written material to customize it specifically for Mrs. Poski.

Action Learning #20: Re-THINKING Action Learning #18

▷ **Rationale:** Rethinking and modifying previous responses reinforces the fact that thinking is an ongoing process that is always growing. Internalization of knowledge increases as students are provided with time and opportunity to explore the learning of new concepts in more depth.

▷ **Teaching Options:** Consider discussing how students feel about changing or not changing their original answers. How do these feelings encourage or hinder their thinking and effective nursing care?

When teaching in the classroom, students can be polled to compare which responses were or were not changed and why. Questions such as the following might be helpful to stimulate thinking. "Was content knowledge the major factor in changing?" "Was a clearer understanding of personal thinking approaches a factor?" "What usually convinces you to make changes?"

If students are not in a classroom, the instructor could ask them to select the three new responses that best reflect their growing skill in understanding and using their personal thinking approaches. Students could describe how they have used this new knowledge in their clinical setting.

Thinking Log #4

To encourage analysis and synthesis of the information in this chapter the student is asked to accomplish two tasks for this Thinking Log. First, the student needs to understand the basic content of the chapter to be able to formulate questions. This may require a second or third reading of parts or all of the chapter. Students can be encouraged to recognize their own unique learning styles and the pace of learning required to grasp the subject matter effectively. The second task is to reinforce the complementary connections between thinking and writing. By writing out the questions, fuzzy thinking can also be "de-fuzzed" as the student is forced to present ideas in an understandable written question.

Class time could be used to examine the students' questions and provide responses. Students could also be asked to continually refer back to the questions in this Thinking Log, then answer and expand on their questions as they progress through the activities in the text.

Monitoring the types of questions developed by students can also provide the instructor with information on content areas that need more emphasis and the kind of thinking being used to develop the questions. For example, are the questions simply focused on content —"How long does it take to write a care plan?" Or, do the questions demonstrate more in-depth thinking— "What is the best way to deal with data that fit into several clusters?"

5

Nursing Conclusions

Chapter 5 begins to focus thinking on the details of the nursing process, specifically conclusions. The critical role of thinking in developing all nursing conclusions is examined. At this early point in the learning process, it is important for students to appreciate the value and purpose of conclusions. Guidance is provided on how nursing conclusions are developed using all five modes of thinking.

▶ **Key Content Areas**

> Examination of the Purpose of Nursing Conclusions
>
> Discussion of the Characteristics of Nursing Conclusions and Process of Making Nursing Conclusions
>
> Incorporation of All Five Modes of THINK to Develop Nursing Conclusions

▶ **Teaching Objectives**

- Guide students' awareness and knowledge about nursing conclusions: their purpose, their characteristics, and how they are made.
- Promote students' valuing of developing accurate nursing conclusions that can be validated.
- Nurture students' ability to identify their THINK modes used to develop conclusions in general and nursing conclusions.

28 ▼ Nursing Conclusions

Rationale and Teaching Options for Action Learning Exercises

▷▷▷▷▷▷Action Learning #21: Tracking Your Thinking through a Conclusion

▷ **Rationale:** This activity continues to encourage students to identify existing conclusion-making skills by using "thinking" vocabulary to describe their skills in making everyday conclusions. Of equal importance is that students recognize how the significance of the final conclusion affects their thinking during the conclusion-making process. Because the seriousness of making conclusions can produce anxiety, the process can again be used as an opportunity to discuss anxiety-reducing techniques. Such techniques might include taking deep breaths, slowing breathing, taking time out to collect thoughts, and so forth.

▷ **Teaching Options:** In the large or small classroom, students could be selected at random to share their findings. Other students could be asked to identify key aspects of thinking that were used. Students could also be paired or placed in triads to share their findings. The instructor could circulate among students and encourage elaboration or clarification of thinking comments.

It is helpful to encourage students to discuss their feelings related to both their thinking and their attempts to describe their thinking. If students find it difficult to get started, the instructor could role model the process to "get the ball rolling."

Discussion can also center on anxiety surrounding important conclusion-making. Finally, a brief discussion of the relationship between existing thinking and how it will be used with nursing can be productive. This helps students continue to build on their natural learning capacities.

▷▷▷▷▷▷Action Learning #22: Hunch Development

▷ **Rationale:** This activity encourages practice with hunch development and recognition of what a hunch "looks like." It helps students realize that some hunches occur almost spontaneously, whereas others may take more thinking to put the pieces together. The discussion section provides six possible hunches that may or may not match with those identified by students.

▷ **Teaching Options:** Students can be asked to write down the specific pieces of information that were used to make their hunch. If they develop hunches not listed in the book, they can be given credit for thinking beyond the obvious if they can support their thinking.

Students can be encouraged to identify what background information was used to develop hunches, for example, personal or professional experience, classes in sociology or culture, knowledge about the side effects of hypertensive medications, and so forth.

This activity can easily be used in the clinical setting with patient data. Students could present separate case studies or all students could focus on one case study. This latter approach provides for validation of conclusions more easily.

It is important at this point to accept *all* hunches because it encourages divergent thinking and prevents thinking from becoming too narrow in the beginning. Nurturing hunch development significantly reduces premature conclusion-making.

Action Learning #23: Ruling in and Ruling out Hunches

▷ **Rationale:** This activity encourages the student to think about specific information that will help support or negate each hunch. The activity requires use of content knowledge that students may have stored in memory; others may need to use textbooks to find the content knowledge. This process of supporting or negating hunches reinforces the importance of using memory and resources along with thinking to put the pieces together.

▷ **Teaching Options:** Students in a large classroom setting can share their findings with classmates. In a smaller classroom setting, students can work in small groups to identify all the resources needed to fill in the data gaps. Discussion can include considerations of stereotypes, attitudes, values, biases, and misinterpretation of information.

Additional discussions can focus on how hunches are developed and ruled in and ruled out in daily life experiences. For example, consider exploring hunches about why a friend didn't call last night, what your mother really meant when she said, "....," how the detective in the mystery story solves the murder so quickly.

Another approach might be to explore with students their natural affinity to make hunches. Do they make many hunches or do they usually stop after the first one pops into their heads? A discussion of the implications of these two different approaches in nursing can be beneficial to beginning students.

This activity is well suited for the clinical setting by using patient data. Helping students see how the instructor thinks to rule in or rule out during a patient care situation is invaluable learning.

▷▷▷▷▷▷Action Learning #24: KNOWING HOW YOU THINK about Ambiguity

▷ **Rationale:** This activity encourages students to self-examine their current comfort level in tolerating conditions that have "answers" relative to the context of the situation rather than simply being right or wrong. Because many students are dualistic in their thinking, they find nursing's high level of ambiguity difficult to deal with. Many students are near graduation before they realize the divergence of their thinking and that required in nursing. Therefore, this exercise, early in their careers, can be most beneficial.

▷ **Teaching Options:** If done in the classroom, students could share and compile their rankings and establish a class range and mean. Discussion about the ability to change comfort levels and what is necessary to make those changes may be appropriate.

This is a good time to help students recognize that many college students are dualistic in their thinking patterns but that doesn't mean they cannot change. Change is more likely to occur with the increased use of the KNOWING HOW YOU THINK mode.

If students are working independently or in a large group they can be encouraged to track their ambiguity tolerance levels over the period of the course, the year, or the nursing program. They could also be encouraged to document for themselves what events or circumstances led to changes in their levels of comfort.

In the clinical setting, students might be encouraged to find patient situations that demonstrate the need to tolerate ambiguity. They could be encouraged to describe patient data that cannot be analyzed using only textbook information and encouraged to discuss how they feel when the patient data do not fit into neat categories.

▷▷▷▷▷▷Action Learning #25: KNOWING HOW YOU THINK and Developing Conclusions

▷ **Rationale:** This activity is designed to help students think more deeply about their thinking styles. It has some repetition with #21 because repetition encourages better integration of learning.

▷ **Teaching Options:** If students are completing this book independently, they can simply follow the directions for sharing their responses with a classmate.

In the classroom setting, small groups of students can share or the class can discuss this exercise as a group. Of particular importance is the student's response to the "why" part of the question. Answering the "why" questions promotes a clearer understanding of thinking. Because "why" questions can be threatening, it is useful for instructors to be aware of the anxiety that may develop. Instructors can remind students that this is a time for learning, all ideas are appropriate, and there are no right or wrong answers.

If students rate themselves as making conclusions without much thinking, it is helpful for the instructor to explore if this is an approach the student thinks will be useful in nursing. Classmates can offer suggestions as to how to nurture an approach that includes more thought.

In the clinical setting, these same questions can be applied to a nursing care assignment. If the students are comfortable with sharing, a postconference group discussion could provide valuable peer input.

Thinking Log #5

Integration of learning occurs best when the student is able to reexamine previous activities and modify them according to new concepts. This Thinking Log allows for the application of the new concepts and development of ownership of the concepts. The student is also asked to summarize the positive skills that are already being used. By building on existing skills (strengths), students are encouraged to learn more.

Class time for classmate sharing can be used to reinforce the learning and to learn from others.

6

Major Nursing Conclusions of Assessment

Chapter 6 focuses on the major nursing conclusions of assessment. Those conclusions are the foundation for nursing care within the remainder of the nursing process. Helping students recognize what they are striving for with assessment helps them appreciate the importance of accurate data collection. Too often, assessment can be perceived by students as collecting and recording that data on a piece of paper. When the conclusion part of assessment is studied first, the act of data collection can take on a broader, more realistic meaning. Teaching strategies in this chapter highlight the thinking processes needed to develop accurate conclusions of assessment.

▶ **Key Content Areas**

    Descriptions of the Major Nursing Conclusions of Assessment—Strengths and Health Concerns

    Differences among the Three Categories of Health Concerns: Nursing Diagnoses, Interdisciplinary Problems, and Problems for Referral

    Differences among Nursing Diagnoses—Actual Problems, Wellness Responses, and Potential Problems

Major Nursing Conclusions of Assessment

▶ Teaching Objectives

- Help students describe the major conclusions of assessment.
- Help students differentiate between nursing diagnoses, interdisciplinary problems, and problems for referral.
- Help students differentiate between actual problems, wellness responses, and potential problems.
- Promote an appreciation of the importance of conclusion-making in assessment.

Rationale and Teaching Options for Action Learning Exercises

▷▷▷▷▷▷Action Learning #26: Finding Patient Strengths

▷ **Rationale:** This activity allows students to expand on their understanding of strengths. It encourages them to think about strengths, figure out why something is a strength, examine feelings about looking for strengths, recognize that strengths are "in the eyes of the beholder," and identify the difficulties in identifying strengths.

▷ **Teaching Options:** This classroom activity can easily be done with a patient in the clinical setting or when collecting data about a classmate's health.

Discussion about one's natural tendency to ignore strengths and generally focus on weaknesses is a good way to start. Students can be asked to list their own strengths and discuss how easy or challenging this task is. One approach would be to examine issues of self-concept and why it might be difficult to identify strengths. For example, it is not uncommon to have received many childhood messages that focused on what they need to do to be "better" rather that acknowledging strengths and growth. Remnants of those early messages frequently remain in the minds of adults and hinder a person's ability to acknowledge strengths.

Discussion could also address the difference between medicine and nursing in that medicine is problem and disease oriented, whereas nursing is focused on the whole person, including the parts that are working well. Emphasis can again be made that the patient's strengths are used to enhance care and design individualized care.

Action Learning #27: Identifying Wellness Diagnoses

▷ **Rationale:** This activity encourages students to think and make judgments as to whether or not a label sounds like a wellness issue or a problem issue. It also helps them recognize that the nursing profession has not studied this area thoroughly. By seeing the profession in progress, students can begin to move from a dualistic style of thinking to a relativistic one in which they can have a significant role in the present and future directions of the profession.

▷ **Teaching Options:** This same activity could be done with any list of nursing diagnoses or nursing issues. Students could also be asked to discuss their feelings about identifying patient wellness responses. It is useful for students to realize that there continues to be considerable debate in this area. This awareness reinforces relativistic versus dualistic thinking. Students could be asked to do a literature search or review the writings in the proceedings of the NANDA conferences to get a better picture of the issues related to wellness.

A clinical focus could include identifying all wellness diagnoses for their assigned patient. Another clinical activity could include interviewing nursing personnel in various settings to determine how often they use wellness diagnoses. A comparison could be made to determine in which settings wellness diagnoses were most prevalent.

Action Learning #28: Differentiating Actual from High-Risk Problems

▷ **Rationale:** This activity allows students to apply what they have learned about actual and high-risk problems to mini data bases. Application increases integration of knowledge because thinking is needed to sort and categorize. The second purpose of this activity is to encourage students to use the resources available in textbooks and again use collaboration as a way of validating and enhancing learning.

▷ **Teaching Options:** Students could be asked to identify at least three texts that support each of their conclusions. Or they could be assigned to find a recent article to support their conclusions and another to negate their conclusions.

Students could discuss a recent clinical patient data base and their conclusions regarding actual and potential problems. It is also helpful to encourage students to describe aloud the thinking that brought them to their conclusions. Discussing differences of opinion about actual and potential problems and having students support their viewpoints promotes peer collaboration and learning.

▷▷▷▷▷▷Action Learning #29: Becoming Familiar with Labels, Definitions, and Defining Characteristics

▷ **Rationale:** This activity allows students to become comfortable with the nursing diagnoses texts used in their particular programs. The more familiarity students have with written material on nursing diagnoses, the more they realize what is available and how they might use the information.

The second purpose of this activity is to familiarize students with the language of nursing diagnoses, what the diagnoses mean, and how to support the diagnoses with the defining characteristics. Exposure to and thinking about the labels, the definitions, and the defining characteristics increase the probability that students will seek accurate conclusions.

▷ **Teaching Options:** Students could be asked to select one new diagnosis each week to share with a classmate. This is an appropriate activity for either the classroom or the clinical setting.

Another possible activity is to have students find five different sources for nursing diagnoses and compare the similarities and differences among the definitions and defining characteristics of each source. Thinking can be nurtured by encouraging them to discuss the reasons for the differences.

Still another activity is to have students prepare a lesson plan to teach another health professional about nursing diagnoses labels, definitions, and defining characteristics. Consider having the students share the outcomes with the class. Teaching is a great way to really learn.

▷▷▷▷▷▷Action Learning #30: Finding an Appropriate Diagnostic Label for Thuscilla

▷ **Rationale:** The major purpose of this activity is to further apply the concepts learned in this and previous chapters. This activity encourages the student to identify important data, cluster the data, think about what the data mean, and identify a diagnostic label that best fits the data. Thinking about, applying, and integrating several of the concepts learned to date are required. Sharing conclusions with a classmate promotes thinking because the student needs to justify conclusions that were made.

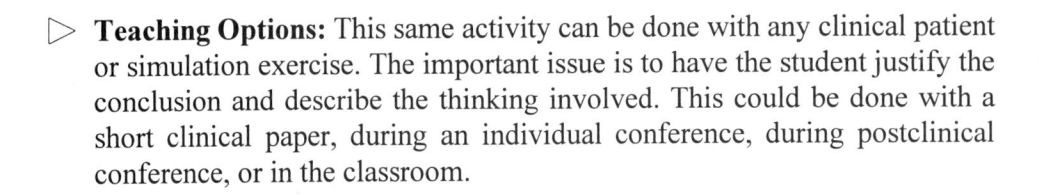

▷ **Teaching Options:** This same activity can be done with any clinical patient or simulation exercise. The important issue is to have the student justify the conclusion and describe the thinking involved. This could be done with a short clinical paper, during an individual conference, during postclinical conference, or in the classroom.

Thinking Log #6

This Thinking Log is designed to engage the student's multiple senses in the learning process. As students translate what was learned through reading into visual images, they must think about and integrate ideas.

A personal creation also instills ownership in the learning process and increases the potential for retention. Sharing the diagram with a classmate requires collaboration and teaching, which increase retention. If the diagram is missing key elements or if it does not fit with the concepts taught, the student can be guided to reexamine, clarify, adjust, or modify. Some helpful words of encouragement such as, "That's a great start; have you considered how you would convey the idea of ...," might be used. This type of comment may be seen as more constructive than critical.

7

Health Detectives: Data Collection and Data Analysis

Chapter 7 focuses on details of assessment and presents a unique approach to data collection that emphasizes how thinking accompanies the task of obtaining information about patients. Many of the ideas presented here can be easily integrated with most health assessment classes and texts and used to augment such courses or texts.

The "detective" idea of collecting data makes use of students' existing knowledge. Who hasn't read about or seen depictions of detectives? Detectives don't just collect information; they constantly think about the relevance of the information and the relationship of each piece of information to other information. The Who, What, Where, When, How, and Why themes are also familiar to most persons and continue the detective analogy throughout the chapter.

This chapter frequently refers to conclusions as discussed in the previous chapters as the purpose of detective work. This continues to reinforce content presented earlier. In addition, links are made to future chapters where content is presented in more detail.

Health Detectives: Data Collection and Data Analysis

▶ Key Content Areas

The Who, What, Where, When, How and Why of Data Collection and Data Analysis

The Thinking and the Doing of Data Collection and Data Analysis

▶ Teaching Objectives

- Encourage constant thinking to accompany data collection and discourage habitual data collection, where data are merely recorded on a form.
- Promote multisensory learning of data collection and data analysis.
- Emphasize how simultaneous data analysis during data collection makes sense and promotes quality assessment.

Rationale and Teaching Options for Action Learning Exercises

Action Learning #31: Distinguishing Types of Data and Inferences

▷ **Rationale:** This activity forces students to think and make a judgment about data. They learn that not all data are straight facts and that some data can only be described as inferences. All too often texts present this distinction between data and inferences dualistically, without presenting the gray areas between inferences and raw data, which are the "necessary inferences."

Part two of the activity takes the thinking a step further so that students will start to think beyond the individual piece of information to combining it with other pieces of information. Introducing the concept of examining one piece of data as it relates to another piece nurtures the understanding of moving toward conclusions during data collection. Unless students see that data are all related to other data, they can easily fall into the trap of collecting data without thinking about their relevance to patients' overall needs.

Part three reinforces students' metacognition skills. Describing their thinking helps students clarify their thought processes.

▷ **Teaching Options:** Obviously, many additional examples could be added to the list given in the text. Students could develop lists themselves and share them with each other. Actual data from clinical situations could be used.

More practice with distinguishing subjective and objective data may be needed, depending on how much of this content students get in other courses or texts. To distinguish between subjective and objective data, students could look at a television program with the sound off and identify objective data.

Then they could close their eyes, turn the sound on, and record the subjective data. Going a step further would reinforce the thinking—students could be asked to make conclusions about what was happening in the TV program, first through analyzing the objective data and then the subjective data. They could compare their conclusions and make judgments about what was missing in each case.

Bringing in the assessment tools that students currently use in clinical settings can be helpful. Students could study those tools to determine if subjective and objective data are to be recorded separately, the types of descriptors listed from which they could choose how to record data, and how tools lend themselves to concurrent analysis as data are collected and recorded.

▷▷▷▷▷▷Action Learning #32: Looking for Relevant Data

▷ **Rationale:** This gets students in the habit of looking things up and making determinations about the relevance of data. A frequent frustration of faculty is that students do not integrate content learned in lectures and texts into the clinical arena. However, faculty would be wise to consider if they have ever taught students *how* to do this. By asking students, early on, to make judgments about data they collect, they are more likely to develop habits of using references and integrating content with practice situations.

▷ **Teaching Options:** This exercise could be incorporated into a clinical assignment or a case study from the students' clinical experiences. Students could prepare a list of data from their latest assessment and then list the norms in that area, or one case could be worked on by a group of students.

This activity could be turned around so that a content area from a textbook or from a class lecture could be discussed for its applications to the nursing process. For instance, if the content area is stress reactions and stress management, students could identify what data they would collect from patients and how they would determine if those data were normal relative to what they had learned about stress.

Another option to acquaint students with references and teach them how to use them to make judgments about relevant data is to assign various books and ask students to find the normal data for a particular content area. Comparisons could be made among several sources for the same content so that students could decide the best sources for certain types of information and discuss reasons for differences in sources.

▷▷▷▷▷ Action Learning #33: Testing Environmental Awareness

▷ **Rationale:** This is a fun activity using everyday situations. Beginning students often get stuck in the asking questions mode of data collection and do not rely on environmental cues as much as they could or should. This activity reinforces the use of other senses besides speech and hearing for collecting data.

This exercise also reinforces the ideas about differentiating raw data and inferences. Discussions of this exercise can show students how some people make inferences about certain things, whereas others can focus on the raw data and distinguish them from inferences.

▷ **Teaching Options:** Variations on this theme could be used. All students could be assigned to watch the same program. Then they could compare notes to see who had picked up on what and how their data collection differed in terms of the raw data and the inferences. Students could give each other feedback on how well they are doing distinguishing raw data from inference or how complete their lists of observations were.

Another tactic that achieves a similar learning outcome is to, unannounced, walk to the back of the room (yourself or ask a student to do it) and ask students to write answers to questions such as, "What color is my (his or her) jacket?" "Does it have lapels?" "Am I wearing glasses?" "Are my teeth straight?" and so forth. This type of activity is usually rich fodder for discussion and humorous teaching. It is often surprising to students to see how observant they are or are not.

▷▷▷▷▷ Action Learning #34: Collecting the DETAIL Clues on a Headache

▷ **Rationale:** DETAIL is another mnemonic that students can easily remember and use in clinical situations. Although most experienced nurses do this detail work almost automatically, beginners need reminders. Using the headache case gives students a common health problem to work with and to which all can relate. Who has never had a headache? Because headaches are different from person to person, students can see how valuable it is to get the details to distinguish the type of headache. Without the DETAIL answers, most beginners might get the same information and make a less precise conclusion of "headache." It is useful to remind students that the data collected to describe the headache will narrow the possible causes and thus incidate the most effective intervention(s).

▷ **Teaching Options:** Use of DETAIL could be demonstrated by a teacher in class so students could see how the questions might be asked. This assignment could be focused on a clinical case with which students are familiar. However, if students are asked to immediately apply the DETAIL to their clinical work, it is important for them to do at least one identical case. Then they can compare notes and see if they are getting the same data, a useful validity and reliability check.

▷▷▷▷▷▷ Action Learning #35: Using Observation Skills

▷ **Rationale:** The rationale for this activity may seem self-evident to most faculty members. Being asked to describe what you see emphasizes that observation is equally valuable to verbal questioning for data collection. In addition to the obvious rationale, this activity gives students an opportunity to collect observed data in a nonthreatening situation, using a picture or a painting. Learning occurs best when students have low anxiety. Often, in situations with patients, students are more anxious and feel uncomfortable just looking at the patient. If they are talking, they are usually so focused on what they and the patient are saying that they do not focus on what they can observe. They can stare as long as they want or need to when the object of study is inanimate.

▷ **Teaching Options:** To show students how naturally they use their observational skills, this activity could be done in class with a timer used to set limits on how long each picture can be observed. Some students see many things quickly; others need extended study to pick up on information. After doing the exercise as a timed activity, students could compare notes on their observations and then share the techniques they use to observe the picture. Some might move their eyes in certain directions; others may think of something like nutrition, activity, or sleep categories to help them look for certain health-related data.

If time allows, faculty could take their class to an art museum to do this exercise. Students could be asked to observe for many things in the works of art, not just health-related information. They might be asked to make a conclusion about what a person in a painting is feeling and then explain their conclusion by listing the raw data that made them think that. Students could look at abstract works of art and describe what they see, what they conclude, and why they drew such conclusions. As long as this exercise is done in a nonthreatening manner where students who know nothing about art feel free to describe their observations, this can be an enriching experience on many levels. If a trip to a museum is not realistic, consider borrowing some slides from the Art Department or use an art history textbook.

▷▷▷▷▷▷Action Learning #36: Practicing Your Measurement Skills

▷ **Rationale:** Besides the obvious value of having students actually practice using instruments, this activity can counteract some of the poor measurement habits they are likely to see in clinical situations. Many nurses can "eyeball" things they have measured many times in the past and estimate quite precisely. Beginning students, on the other hand, who have never seen a decubitus ulcer before, much less measured one, cannot expect to be as accurate in their estimates.

One of the most important aspects of this activity is for students to see the value in precise data collection and to value measurement. The discussion, as guided by the questions in the text, is extremely important. Often students are told to measure things, but they fail to see the value in such detail work because they have not been taught *why* such precision is important. Bringing in case examples of patients with ascites (where changes in abdominal girth are vital to determining patient progress or decline) or discovering a patient's deep vein thrombosis (where increased leg circumference is critical) or other such examples can show students the value of measurement quite graphically.

▷ **Teaching Options:** Instructors will likely want to use measurement examples that are relevant to the student's clinical setting while they are completing this text. Students could be assigned specific things to measure that are most relevant to their clinical population.

This exercise could be done as a fun game. Props could be used so that each student has a different "condition." Cards with vague descriptions of those conditions could be distributed. Then students would find the person with the "matching condition" on his or her card, measure what had been vaguely described or shown in the props, and write out a new description. Washable body paint can be used to make a rash for the person who has a "small rash on body." A pillow in someone's sleeve would make a "left arm smaller than the right." The "actual" temperature of a person drinking a hot beverage would replace the vague description of "elevated temperature." Black wax on teeth can allow for an accurate count of "some teeth missing." A scale could be used to measure the person who is "very thin," but to keep discomfort down, it's best not to use the opposite example—"very large." The examples used would only be restricted by the instructor's imagination.

Thinking Log #7

This log reinforces the content presented in this chapter by asking students to review what they learned. Because the content of this chapter has direct application in clinical situations, the directions ask students to do more than remember, but to think about how they can apply the things they have learned. This focus on application should again help students integrate content with practice.

This log also focuses on metacognition, which helps students identify and describe their best ways of learning. By now, halfway through the text, instructors may want to pay particular attention to how well students are able to describe their thinking about their thinking. Those students who are still focused on *what* they are thinking more than *how* they are thinking may need additional assistance with their metacognition skills.

8

Making More Sense of Clues: Cluster Analysis

This chapter is a continuation of the analysis of data started in Chapter 7. Vital to the thinking necessary for accurate conclusion-making, cluster analysis helps students deal with large amounts of information using the brain's natural memory systems. Cluster analysis helps students see data gaps and the importance of filling in those gaps. It also shows them how to form clusters and to understand the significance of the clusters to the final conclusions of assessment.

Teaching strategies aimed at helping students use their natural thinking patterns are helpful to learning this process. Instructors thinking out loud as they demonstrate analysis of data clusters will be helpful to students.

▶ **Key Concepts**

Clusters from an Actual Patient Data Base

Thinking during Cluster Analysis

Making More Sense of Clues: Cluster Analysis   45

▶ Teaching Objectives

- Promote an appreciation of the importance of clusters to forming conclusions.
- Help students form clusters from data bases.
- Maintain an openness to cluster analysis so that individual thinking styles can be used optimally.

Rationale and Teaching Options for Action Learning Exercises

▷▷▷▷▷▷Action Learning #37: Looking for "Point B"

▷ **Rationale:** This exercise capitalizes on the student's natural thinking sequences. Before "Point B" is explained in the text or by an instructor, students can develop their own thoughts about it. The case study is fairly simple so students should not get caught up in a medical situation that may be foreign to them. Because students are asked to think of other possible conclusions, they are given a message that all possible answers are not necessarily given in printed texts. Such a lesson in relativistic thinking is part of the continuing message of learning exercises in this book.

▷ **Teaching Options:** Obviously other case studies could be used to a similar end. For students who are in a clinical setting, their cases could be analyzed. It might be helpful if all students use the same case at least once so that they can see how alternative conclusions and clusters are possible.

The questions in the discussion section can provide a start for rich discussions of recording formats for data, various assessment tools, or other methods of relaying information about patients. This case was purposefully presented in a somewhat mixed-up sequence so that such discussion would ensue. Pieces of information about various patient responses are spread throughout the description.

▷▷▷▷▷▷Action Learning #38: Examining Clusters

▷ **Rationale:** Showing clusters by themselves outside of a patient situation allows a "clean" look at clusters without extraneous information. This lets students tap into their natural brain patterns and think about why these clusters do or do not make sense to them. The significant clusters represent familiar patterns that beginners are likely to have experienced—A is a cold, C is constipation, D is anxiety or stress. The data in clusters B and E are obviously nonclusters. A discussion could address why they are nonclusters. Working with these common clusters and nonclusters can show students that clustering is something they deal with in everyday life.

▷ **Teaching Options:** Clearly, many similar clusters could be developed. Students could describe a cluster of symptoms they have experienced and see if the class can label it. They could use examples from their clinical work. It is best not to make the clusters too complicated at this point until the whole group understands the essential structure of clusters.

▷▷▷▷▷▷Action Learning #39: Looking for Data Gaps

▷ **Rationale:** This exercise is important to students' full thinking repertoire. It is often glossed over in traditional texts that give full data clusters as explanations of nursing phenomena. Thinking about data that are not there is as important as, if not more important than, thinking about what data are there.

The hint about using textbooks to help with this activity guides students to integrate the content knowledge necessary to making judgments about missing data. Encouraging use of resources lets students know that they are not expected to automatically know this sophisticated aspect of thinking.

▷ **Teaching Options:** Other clusters, perhaps relevant to other content areas being studied simultaneously, could be used instead of or in addition to the clusters presented in the text. A fun approach to this learning is to use role playing. A student could give symptoms of not feeling well, leaving out critical information, to see if the class can ask the necessary questions to get at the missing information. A reminder to use DETAIL may also be helpful.

▷▷▷▷▷▷Action Learning #40: Tapping Your Life Experience

▷ **Rationale:** A recurrent theme in this text is to have students use existing knowledge and thinking skills and then apply them to nursing situations. This exercise removes the unfamiliar qualities of patient situations and helps students think about what they already know. It is nonthreatening and helps them appreciate their existing knowledge and thinking abilities. Reinforcement of earlier learning about the differences between objective and subjective data (signs and symptoms) is also part of this exercise. Repetition enhances learning.

▷ **Teaching Options:** This exercise could be done in a classroom setting. A round-robin discussion could be used with questions such as: "When you are tired, what do you feel like?" "When you are under stress, what happens?"

Each student could add signs or symptoms to these familiar scenarios. A secondary purpose of increasing students' awareness of what it feels like to be a patient could be met if they are asked to list probable feelings and perceptions of sick people. Answers to this question could produce data that could be studied as a cluster: "If you were a patient, what would you be feeling?"

Action Learning #41: Using the Assessment Tool to Find Preliminary Clusters

▷ **Rationale:** Using an assessment tool to help with data clustering gives added meaning to the use of tools. Too often tools are seen as pieces of paper on which information is simply recorded; they are not viewed as aids to thinking, clustering data, and analyzing the clusters. The tool in this text is one based on the NANDA taxonomic structure and can reinforce clustering that leads to nursing diagnosis conclusions.

▷ **Teaching Options:** Assessment tools are individualized within many nursing curricula. Obviously, if students are using a different tool, they would want to use that in this exercise. As many faculty will attest, the NANDA taxonomic structure is sometimes cumbersome when applied to an assessment tool. However, in keeping with our attempts to be consistent with the NANDA work, the tool in this book was arranged with NANDA's scheme as an organizing system.

Discussions of this exercise could include a consideration of different forms of tools. This discussion will be particularly helpful in this context if it focuses on how various tools help with clustering data so that nursing conclusions can be made. Using clinical examples where data were recorded on a tool will be helpful to students' learning. They can indicate where the clusters naturally "fall out" and where they are more obscure or disjointed. Because patient data rarely fit into neat boxes, the importance of thinking beyond the natural clustering found in tools usually emerges as students ask questions about data analysis.

Action Learning #42: Another Look at Clusters for Actual and Potential Problems

▷ **Rationale:** This exercise has some elements that are a repetition of an Action Learning exercise in Chapter 6. That repetition is important to learning something as complex as data clusters. In addition to recognizing clusters, this exercise promotes the use of resources to help make conclusions about clusters. This activity promotes the integration of theoretical and clinical content.

Determining potential problems is often difficult for beginning students who have limited content knowledge to know the risk factors in a patient situation. With this additional information on clustering, the differences between actual and potential problem clusters should become more evident.

▷ **Teaching Options:** This exercise could be done in class or in small groups. Students could compare the wording of their conclusions and share the resources they used. Another classroom teaching method is to play a matching game. Clusters and cluster labels, each written on separate cards, are mixed up. Different colors can be used for potential and actual problems. Students then work in small groups or individually to make the best matches.

▷▷▷▷▷▷Action Learning #43: Selecting the Best Label

▷ **Rationale:** This exercise helps students use reference materials in a meaningful way. The fine differences among the labels given in the exercise can help students avoid choosing the most obvious label. This discrimination of finer differences is not presented in most nursing textbooks; often clusters are linked with only one label. If the "one cluster—one label" approach is all that students are exposed to, they can be misled into believing that choosing a label is a dualistic, either/or action, devoid of much thought.

Most faculty can relate to the frustration of grading clinical work where students have chosen the most obvious label for a cluster of data and the care plan looks as if it were copied from a book. Not much depth of understanding is apparent in that type of work. However, teaching students how to discriminate so that the most descriptive label is used is challenging. Indeed, it is often not even taught. The extra effort with beginners, however, is well worth it. This effort pays off in increased quality of students' clinical work.

▷ **Teaching Options:** Faculty could use their files of student clinical work and find many examples of nursing diagnoses that were picked without much discriminating thought. Students could analyze those examples and, as a group, discuss how a better label could have been found. It is often easier for students to see how poorly discriminated work can be made better than it is for them to discriminate from the outset themselves.

Thinking Log #8

    This log asks students to pull together information they learned in Chapters 5 through 8, all of which relates to thinking and doing during assessment. It also asks them to relate what they have learned to their personal thinking styles. If class time is available, the students' entries in this log could be shared. It would be helpful to all students to see how others have pulled this complex content together.

9

Designing, Doing, and Determining Quality of Care

a.k.a. Planning, Implementing, and Evaluating

Many faculty may find the approach of this chapter a bit unusual. Often, in nursing texts, planning, implementing, and evaluating are treated as separate entities. However, we believe that valuable connections get lost when the interrelationships of these parts of the process are not addressed. Although it is often acknowledged that the nursing process is not linear, few illustrations are available to students that show *how* relativistic and contextual it actually is. The vivid illustration at the beginning of this chapter should be a reinforcement to readers that using all parts of the nursing process is not a linear set of actions and thought but rather a well-balanced and skilled juggling act.

When planning is learned without a simultaneous consideration of implementing and evaluating, the plan can become a piece of paper only. Thought must consistently focus on how that plan will be carried out for it to be realistic and individualized to the patient. When evaluation is not considered during planning, the importance of well-developed goals and objectives may be obscured.

Another important message of this chapter is the conclusion-making that is as integral to planning, implementing, and evaluating as it is to assessing. The use of alternative terms, such as designing and determining quality, reinforce that judgments are being made in all parts of the nursing process. Determining quality of care, for example, implies that a conclusion about the nature of the care is being made.

▶ Key Content Areas

Connections among Planning, Implementing, and Evaluating

How Conclusions Are Made during Planning, Implementing, and Evaluating

Thinking Used to Design, Do, and Determine Quality of Care

▶ Teaching Objectives

- Promote relativistic thinking during planning, implementing, and evaluating care.
- Help students learn how to plan care that is based on thinking of the "big picture" of the patient situation, not just as a task to produce a piece of paper called a "care plan."

Rationale and Teaching Options for Action Learning Exercises

▷▷▷▷▷▷Action Learning #44: Setting Priorities

▷ **Rationale:** As the text preceding this exercise describes it, setting priorities is not as simple a task as it is often reported to be through use of traditional priority-setting schemes. In this exercise, students can use the complex thinking necessary to effectively set priorities with patients. To reinforce the message that students often can add important insights to what is written in books, this exercise asks students to add diagnoses that they identify as missed in the example. Students will find that it is difficult to set priorities without being able to talk with the patient in this situation. That difficulty is included on purpose to emphasize the importance of this decision being made collaboratively with patients.

▷ **Teaching Options:** Actual patient situations from students' clinical work could be equally or more valuable to learning about setting priorities. It will be especially helpful if students can describe to others how they thought about

52 ▼ Designing, Doing, and Determining Quality of Care

and set priorities. Feedback from other students who may have approached the situation differently will promote an appreciation of alternative, perhaps equally valuable, approaches.

If the text's situation is a focus for class discussion, it may be enriching for students to talk about the influence of their values and beliefs on setting priorities. Mrs. Partridge's decisional conflict about breastfeeding, for example, usually elicits strong beliefs about the value of breastfeeding versus bottle feeding.

▷▷▷▷▷▷Action Learning #45: Establishing Goals

- ▷ **Rationale:** This exercise is fairly straightforward in its intent to give students practice with wording goals that are related to nursing diagnoses. A variety of types of nursing diagnoses are provided so students can see how goals are alike or different depending on the type of diagnosis.
- ▷ **Teaching Options:** Students' clinical diagnoses and plans could be used instead of the examples given in this exercise. Each student could bring in a plan in which it was difficult to establish goals for the patient. Several of these could be chosen and discussed by the whole class. Alternatively, small groups could be set up and all examples from the group could be discussed. Each group could then report to the larger group on what they had learned about establishing goals.

▷▷▷▷▷▷Action Learning #46: Finding Measurable Objectives

- ▷ **Rationale:** Establishing measurable objectives is often difficult for beginning students. When the link to evaluation is made, as it is in this chapter, the relevance of measurability becomes clearer than when objectives are established without thought of their later use in evaluation. The listed objectives are common ones seen in many clinical situations; chances are students have seen similar well-worded and the not-so-well-worded objectives in their clinical sites.
- ▷ **Teaching Options:** Like the previous exercise on goals, examples from students' clinical work could be used as examples to illustrate measurable and nonmeasurable objectives. It may also help students learn the importance of measurability if a classroom analogy is used. For example, students could look at course or lecture objectives developed by faculty and discuss the importance of measurability to their being graded according to those objectives.

▷▷▷▷▷ Action Learning #47: Adding Time Frames

▷ **Rationale:** Time frames are often hard for beginning students to determine because they have little experience on which to draw such conclusions. Having students think about what information they need to know to identify time frames will help them focus on the thinking involved in this activity. Taking this approach discourages students from expecting appropriate time frames to just appear in books or drop out of the sky.

Setting time frames as part of planning also connects planning to evaluating. Without a consideration of planning *and* evaluation, time frames can become relatively meaningless.

▷ **Teaching Options:** This exercise will be richer if real situations from students' clinical work can be used as examples, rather than those in the book. Using real examples can show students how important the whole context of the patient's situation is to setting time frames.

An optimal learning experience would be for students to do the book exercise and then discuss their real patient situations. They can see the differences between an exercise without a context and a contextually defined situation.

▷▷▷▷▷ Action Learning #48: Thinking through to Establishing Objectives to Select the Best Nursing Diagnosis

▷ **Rationale:** This exercise is perhaps one of the most valuable for showing students the interconnectedness of the phases of the nursing process and the nonlinear quality of the process. Few textbook explanations of nursing process go "backward" like this to show how a nursing diagnosis can be better differentiated during the planning phase of care. Yet, it is not uncommon for students to get bogged down in a care plan that doesn't work and spin their wheels for hours. Helping students to reverse their thinking when they get bogged down will refocus their thinking, decrease their frustration, and help them ground their plans in reality.

▷ **Teaching Options:** This is one exercise that we hope all students will do and discuss with instructors. The learning is so valuable that we also hope that instructors take the discussion one step further by asking students to bring in their problem plans and think them through "backward."

Copyright © 1995 J. B. Lippincott Co., Instructor's Manual to Accompany *Critical Thinking in Nursing: An Interactive Approach*

Action Learning #49: Establishing Objectives

▷ **Rationale:** Like #45, where students established goals, this exercise provides practice in establishing objectives. By now they have read about and done exercises on making objectives clear, measurable, and time framed; this exercise allows them to pull all of that together.

▷ **Teaching Options:** Learning will be enhanced if students can have an opportunity to apply this learning to their clinical work. Therefore, if students are concurrently in a clinical setting, it is most helpful if they bring examples of their clinical work to class for further discussion. Objective writing is difficult for most beginners, so repetition with constructive feedback is important.

For students who are not in a clinical setting while they are using this text, nonnursing examples could be used. They could develop objectives for a class topic, vacation, preparation for graduate school, or any other situation.

Action Learning #50: Individualizing a Standardized Care Plan

▷ **Rationale:** Beginning students, as most faculty well know, often are so overwhelmed with learning nursing that they latch on to standard care plans and rewrite them to hand in to their instructors, often without much individualization to the particular patient for whom they are planning care. This exercise helps them focus on the individualization issue. Diversional Activity Deficit was chosen for the nursing diagnosis example because it is personal to people who have that problem.

Having students explain their changes and why they made those changes helps them clarify their thinking about individualization and show how standardized plans are best used to trigger thinking.

▷ **Teaching Options:** One of the questions in the discussion following this exercise is, "If you were the patient, what would you want?" A discussion centered on that question is helpful to students' valuing of individualized care. Role playing patient situations, especially if some reality-promoting props are used, can be beneficial. A student could be assigned the role of a patient with a communication deficit, for example, and given a set of directions for acting out a problem, such as an uncomfortable position in a bed as he or she is turned from side to side by other students. A plan for care could be developed using standard plans for impaired mobility, for example, with all students identifying what should be changed to individualize the plan.

Another tactic, but one that may be delicate in terms of agency diplomacy, is for students to find nonindividualized care plans for patients in their clinical agencies. Those plans could then be individualized. Qualifying statements to students about reasons why nurses might write such plans on patients' records may diffuse some of the "criticism" nuances.

Action Learning #51: What's Missing in This Written Plan?

▷ **Rationale:** This exercise helps students pull together much of what they have learned in this chapter. The repetition will enhance retention of information. Evaluating a plan that is not well done is also less threatening than having to write a plan from scratch using all of the criteria for developing plans.

▷ **Teaching Options:** Students who are concurrently in clinical settings would probably welcome the opportunity to have some feedback on their plans. Therefore, a great learning experience is to have students trade plans with each other and critique the work according to the criteria used to critique the plan in the exercise.

Action Learning #52: Finding Safe, Effective, and Efficient Ways to Implement Nursing Care

▷ **Rationale:** Peer collaboration is important to learning. Having students talk to experienced nurses about their care can promote lifelong habits of collaboration. Practicing nurses often have a slightly different perspective on implementing care than instructors or students have. Much can be learned from nurses who are "out there" every day. By having all students talk to a practicing nurse, many different perspectives can be gathered, which can then be shared with the rest of the class.

▷ **Teaching Options:** This exercise may be difficult if students are not concurrently in a clinical setting. However, many students know a practicing nurse with whom they could talk. An alternative plan is to invite one or several nurses to class and set up a panel discussion of the questions in the exercise.

Action Learning #53: Tracking One's Method of Evaluating

▷ **Rationale:** Because of the schedules in many schools of nursing, it is often difficult for students to fully evaluate care they have implemented. They often get patient assignments, see patients, and then plan care that they may not get to implement. This is particularly the case in acute care settings where patients are often discharged before students can work with them a second time. Therefore, many learning activities, but especially evaluations, are done only as theoretical exercises—''I would evaluate this way,'' rather than ''I evaluated....''

Unfortunately, a text like this one, also must leave evaluation in the theoretical realm unless students are given a specific evaluation exercise to do. This exercise, hopefully, can be done in a clinical context where students can evaluate the actual care they have implemented.

▷ **Teaching Options:** This exercise is best done by having students evaluate their own so that the Evaluation Tracking Patterns method can be used. An alternative approach is offered for students who are not in a clinical setting while they do this exercise. Describing how one evaluated a life event can be beneficial because it relates evaluation in nursing to a process also used in everyday life.

Another exercise would be to give students case studies that include descriptions of nursing care so that they can evaluate the care in the case study. If all students are given the same case, they can compare their evaluation approaches and learn from each other as well.

Thinking Log #9

By now students will likely have made changes in their thinking patterns. In this log they are asked to redraw their thinking caps and describe the changes that have occurred since the first drawing in Chapter 1. This exercise promotes self-reflection (metacognition) and is often rewarding to students. Instructors may want to allow class time for students to describe their revised thinking caps so all students can see the progress made by others. We do not recommend grading this exercise, however, because grading may stifle a student's free expression.

10

Written and Verbal Communication of Thinking and Doing

One chapter on communication barely scratches the surface of what students need to learn about the topic. However, because communication is essential to great nursing, this book would not be complete without at least some acknowledgement of its importance. Hopefully, instructors can link this chapter to other learning opportunities having to do with communication.

The second part of the chapter, which addresses the finer points of communication, is probably unique to this book. Studying the choice of words for describing parts of the nursing process has not been covered in most nursing texts. Yet, most experienced nurses and instructors will likely agree that the thinking and communication described here are, in reality, things that they do regularly. This chapter attempts to whet the appetites of beginning students to these finer points of communication.

▶ **Key Content Areas**

Similarities and Differences between Verbal and Written Communication
Communicating the Thinking and Doing Parts of the Nursing Process
How Subtleties of Communication Can Enhance the Quality of the Nursing Process

58 ▼ Written and Verbal Communication of Thinking and Doing

▶ Teaching Objectives

- Promote an appreciation of the importance of communication as part of the nursing process.
- Provide practice with verbal and written communication techniques.
- Help students communicate their thinking.

Rationale and Teaching Options for Action Learning Exercises

▷▷▷▷▷▷Action Learning #54: Evaluating Your Verbal Communication

▷ **Rationale:** This exercise is meant to graphically show students how they communicate verbally. Because few people have a clear idea how they sound to others, listening to themselves on a tape can be enlightening.

This assignment allows students to communicate about something they know well, which can be less threatening than communicating something about nursing. Allowing students to evaluate their usual methods of speech builds on existing thinking patterns before nursing is introduced.

▷ **Teaching Options:** Many nursing curricula have a built-in communication course or other learning experiences. If this exercise is duplicative of others in the curriculum, obviously, it could be skipped. If nothing comparable is offered, we highly recommend that students complete this exercise.

This exercise could be incorporated with other learning experiences, such as a required presentation on a preset topic. Hopefully, audio or video taping will be used so that students can hear or see themselves.

An alternative experience is to have students identify persons they believe are good communicators and those who are not. They could list the characteristics of each person's speech style and discuss why one is perceived as a better communicator.

▷▷▷▷▷▷Action Learning #55: Evaluating Elie's Communication

▷ **Rationale:** Many instructors may chuckle at the end-of-shift report in this exercise. A bit extreme, it is meant to show students how not to communicate. The illustrations of Elie that accompany this exercise should be a funny visual reminder of what they should and should not aspire to in their communication. Like some others in this book, this exercise shows what not to do so that students can correct the problems in a nonthreatening situation.

Written and Verbal Communication of Thinking and Doing ▼ 59

▷ **Teaching Options:** Students who are concurrently in a clinical setting could practice end-of-shift reports based on their care. They could try to do them incorrectly and then correct them, which often adds humor to the learning experience.

For students who are not in a clinical setting, movies or TV shows depicting nurses could be assigned and students could do an analysis of the communication. Chances are, students will be able to pick up many problematic communication styles doing that exercise.

We encourage use of class time to discuss this exercise. Several questions posed in the discussion section could start such a class. Elie's ideal report is included after the discussion section, so it could be discussed in class also.

▷▷▷▷▷▷ Action Learning #56: Finding the Documentation Errors in a Progress Note

▷ **Rationale:** Although students should be encouraged to develop their personal communication styles using their strengths, a set structure is still needed for writing notes on a patient's record. This exercise helps students apply what they learned in the preceding paragraph about documentation rules. The exercise itself is fairly simple, but a focus on thinking in the discussion section makes it more than just a how-to exercise.

▷ **Teaching Options:** Instructors could add more examples of notes, perhaps those done in other formats, to this exercise. It is often easier for students to see the problems in someone else's notes than to develop well-worded notes themselves. Extra practice will be helpful.

Students in a clinical setting, who have access to medical records, could be asked to keep track of questions they had as they read records. They could then discuss their observations and determine if clarity of communication or some other issue was the root of the problem.

▷▷▷▷▷▷ Action Learning #57: Writing a Narrative Note; #58: Sorting the Parts of a SOAP Note; and #59: Writing a DAR Note

▷ **Rationale:** These three exercises are addressed together because each is a straightforward practice session with a different style of recording. The rationales behind these exercises are likely clear to instructors. Students need practice, lots of it, with writing chart notes. These three formats are offered as examples because they are commonly found in health care settings. Giving students opportunities to write notes in nonthreatening settings outside of clinical situations will help them engage their higher level thinking while learning these techniques.

▷ **Teaching Options:** Obviously, if another style of charting is used in the students' clinical agencies, practice with that format should be added to or substituted for the formats in these exercises. Additional case studies also could be used to reinforce this learning.

Thinking Log #10

This log, like several other exercises and logs, asks students to look at the world of nursing practice and learn from it. Instructors may want to discuss this assignment before students do it so that everyone is clear on the intent—that it is not to find problems with other nurses' records, but to see a variety of written communication styles and learn from that experience. Although probably unnecessary to state, it is assumed that all exercises that involve patient records will be dealt with in a strictly confidential manner, without patients' names attached to any material written about clinical situations. Students may need periodic reminders of this important issue throughout their work with this book.

11

Consequences of Thinking and Not Thinking When Documenting

This chapter introduces a bit of shock treatment into students' learning about thinking and communication. Written by a nurse who both practices nursing and consults as an expert witness in health care litigation, the case examples in this chapter were selected to show students, in no uncertain terms, the consequences of thinking and not thinking. This chapter also reviews all phases of the nursing process to show how thinking and documentation of that thinking are integrated. To enhance retention of content learned earlier, some content is repeated. New information builds on that previous learning.

This chapter's author has been a guest lecturer to our students while they are studying this book. Students have engaged in hours of lively discussion about quality care and legal issues. If the content of this chapter can be linked to other such content in the curriculum, learning is greatly enhanced. Instructors may want to look at their curriculum content on legal, ethical, and quality assurance topics and make links to the thinking focus of this chapter and this text.

Key Content Areas

The Relationship of Nursing Process, Thinking, Documentation, Quality Assurance, and Legal Issues

Case Studies Illustrating Problematic Thinking and Use of the Nursing Process

Teaching Objectives

- Promote a value of clear documentation that reflects thinking, quality assurance, and legal accountability.
- Help students appreciate the seriousness of high-quality documentation.

Rationale and Teaching Options for Action Learning Exercises

Action Learning #60: Mr. Schultz's Missing Care; #61: Mr. Fodler's Missing Care

▷ **Rationale:** These two exercises are discussed together because of their similarity. By now, students have had repeated exposure to parts of the nursing process. These case studies and others in this chapter are a test of that learning. Specific, directed questions help students zero in on the specific areas of the process that are missing. Other questions also help students imagine how they would feel in the patient's place. This self-reflection enhances a student's sensitivity to the unique feelings of patients.

▷ **Teaching Options:** Most instructors have a wide repertoire of case studies such as these that they could use to reinforce learning. Instructors may choose to substitute studies more closely linked to students' particular clinical area of focus if these medical-surgical examples seem inappropriate to the students' level of knowledge.

Action Learning #62: Analyzing Documentation for Mrs. Hendricks; #63: Analyzing Documentation for Ms. Rose, Parts A, B, & C

▷ **Rationale:** The documentation examples in these exercises show sets of notes by several nurses with regard to two patients. Students often do not consider ramifications of shift changes on continuity of care in hospitals, so these examples add a different perspective. Students can see that what one nurse does is often influenced by what others do. Hopefully they will begin to appreciate the fact that each nurse must be personally accountable for all parts of the nursing process. Again, analyzing someone else's notes often produces less anxiety than writing a note. The discussion questions bring in the legal perspective as students are asked to picture themselves as lawyers defending the nurses who wrote the notes. Thought of legal defense of one's work is often a startling, but effective (eye-opening) form of learning.

▷ **Teaching Options:** As with the previous two exercises, other examples more related to students' current clinical area of study could be used instead of the examples here. To reinforce the focus on legal issues, instructors may want to invite a nurse-attorney or a nurse who does legal work to talk with students about this and other documentation examples.

▷▷▷▷▷▷Action Learning #64: Charting Patient Responses and Nursing Care

▷ **Rationale:** This exercise shows students qualitative differences in notes by nurses who may both have given similar care. The first note does not describe patient responses but the second one does. The fine distinctions of what should be included in a note is both a review of content from Chapter 10 and an opportunity to consider other issues. Students can compare and contrast poorly written notes to well written ones and see the differences.

▷ **Teaching Options:** The objective of this exercise can be met with examples of nursing notes. Students could analyze notes that they have written or share several examples that a whole class could analyze. Specific content areas being learned in other concurrent classes could be incorporated into examples of notes to reinforce other learning as well.

▷▷▷▷▷▷Action Learning #65: Mr. Smock's Missing Details

▷ **Rationale:** Students usually do not get a chance to participate in a quality assurance audit. Putting oneself in the shoes of an auditor can provide a new perspective on documentation.

▷ **Teaching Options:** The intent of this exercise would be accomplished even more fully if students could participate in an actual chart audit in a clinical agency. Some instructors may be able to arrange such an experience. They could also be assigned a task to find audit criteria in an agency and use those criteria to judge some of their own notes or those of other students.

Action Learning #66: Tracking an Incident: Mr. Katz's IV

▷ **Rationale:** The legal ramifications of incidents and incident reporting are important aspects of professional nursing. Students will likely receive additional information on this subject in other courses, so this exercise and its accompanying discussion are merely a quick overview. However, even beginning students must understand and appreciate the relevance of thinking within the framework of the nursing process when it comes to incident reports.

▷ **Teaching Options:** Ideally, students will be able to find incident reports in their clinical agencies and practice writing notes such as the one in this exercise. Each agency has its own rules relating to incidents, so it is expected that instructors would individualize this learning experience to their agencies and their curricula.

Thinking Log #11

Depending on how many additional examples of notes an instructor has used to augment the exercises in this chapter, this log may or may not be redundant. If students have just done the exercises as described, this log will be a valuable learning experience to help them solidify the content of this chapter. Anticipating an involvement in legal action may produce anxiety for some students, so it is helpful if some discussion of this topic can be planned for class time.

12

Assessing a Complete Patient Situation

Chapter 12 begins the final section of the text. This last segment returns the student to the "big picture" of great nursing. With the use of a more complex case study and a checklist to track thinking, these final chapters document the integration of content knowledge, thinking skills, and the nursing process.

Chapter 12 focuses specifically on assessment, the major conclusions of assessment, and priority setting with the patient. This chapter provides the foundation on which great nursing care can be planned, implemented, and evaluated in the succeeding chapters.

The case study for these last chapters was selected because it provided an opportunity for students to learn from more complex nursing care in a home care setting. It provides opportunities for students to "see" the nurse's thinking while they continue to practice using the concepts learned in earlier chapters. Use of newly learned concepts with gradually increasing complexity provides internalization of learning and recognition of how nursing care needs to be "tweaked" here and there to fit each unique patient situation.

▶ **Key Content Areas**

Return to the "Big Picture" of Great Nursing after Reviewing the Details
Introduce the Tracking Nursing Thinking (TNT) Checklist
Introduce the Case Study to be Used for the Final Chapters

Assessing a Complete Patient Situation

Examine the Thinking Skills, Content Knowledge, and Nursing Process Skills Used to Develop the Major Conclusions of Assessment and Set Priorities

▶ Teaching Objectives

- Help students recognize the concepts they have been learning as those concepts are applied to a more complex case study.
- Provide more opportunities for practice and repetition with constant reminders to blend the details with the "big picture."
- Guide use of the TNT Checklist.

Rationale and Teaching Options for Action Learning Exercises

▷▷▷▷▷▷ Action Learning #67: Identifying Possible Sources for Content Knowledge Needed to Prepare for Data Collection with Betty

▷ **Rationale:** This activity is designed to help students recognize and acknowledge that it takes time and patience to learn what content knowledge is needed before caring for a patient. A secondary purpose is to encourage students to seek multiple sources of information, discover the differences in information, and discuss the reasons for the differences.

▷ **Teaching Options:** Class discussion could include an exploration of the types of sources and their differences, differences related to older versus more current sources, differences between information in journal articles versus text books, policy manuals, or expert nurses.

If this activity is done as a clinical project, students could be asked to locate sources of information relative to their assigned patients rather than the case study or in addition to the case study.

No matter what the setting, it is helpful for students to share with peers the techniques they use to streamline the process of acquiring content knowledge. Some students, for example, might discuss how they use a book index, references at the end of articles, computer searches, or textbooks from other courses such as pathophysiology or abnormal psychology. This is a good time to remind students to save care plans and develop some methods of keeping track of useful sources for future references.

▷▷▷▷▷▷Action Learning #68: What Are Your First Impressions?

▷ **Rationale:** Continued practice and repetition of concepts learned in earlier chapters increases retention of learning. This activity again allows students to draw on their expanding thinking skills and continue to mold those skills into effective ways to approach nursing care.

Divergent thinking is the focus here, nurturing INQUIRY and NEW IDEAS AND CREATIVE THINKING to elicit as many first impressions as possible. Studies indicate that most diagnostic errors occur because the accurate diagnosis was never considered as an option to be ruled in or ruled out.

This activity also acknowledges the initial feelings of being overwhelmed with the complexity of the situation. It encourages the student to deal with those feelings by looking for relationships among the data, looking for clusters, and making the volume of data more manageable.

▷ **Teaching Options:** This same activity can be used in any setting or with any set of data, simulations, case studies, or real clinical patients. The primary objective is to stimulate thinking and creativity. This can be done by suggesting some far-fetched first impressions to "prime the pump." In a class setting, writing all first impressions on the board without critique or challenge will help students feel less anxious about volunteering their ideas.

The instructor could also ask each student to write ideas on paper and then call on each student to share one idea to be written on a board. At the end of the allotted time period, students could be encouraged to add any additional ideas that had not already been addressed.

After the divergent thinking ideas have been shared, a discussion could focus on convergent thinking. The instructor could ask: "How did these impressions occur?" "What data can be used to support these impressions?" "Which first impressions need more attention?" "How did clustering and seeing patterns help with first impressions?" "How did the TNT tool help or hinder?" "How will the first impressions affect the rest of data collection?"

All of these questions and others could be used to encourage the students' thinking. It will be helpful if the instructor continues to reward the evidence of thinking as well as the outcomes of thinking.

▷▷▷▷▷Action Learning #69: Validating Hunches

▷ **Rationale:** This activity is a natural continuation of the thinking begun with first impressions. The objective now is to fine tune conclusions and increase the probability of accuracy.

The questions provided in the text encourage additional practice for students in using written resources to make matches between data and current theory or diagnostic labels. These questions promote thinking beyond the simple matching to find stronger support for their hunches. The final question concerning differential diagnosis is used to stimulate divergent thinking again. Helping students recognize the constant flow between divergent and convergent thinking provides a valuable understanding of the full repertoire of thinking skills needed for great nursing.

▷ **Teaching Options:** This activity can be done in any setting using this case study or another. Answers to the questions posed in the text could be required with all written care plans. Instructors could ask these questions of students in the clinical setting to assess their ability to develop accurate nursing diagnoses before planning care.

In the large classroom, students could work for short periods of time in small groups and share their results with the whole class. Discussion could center around the similarities and differences in the validation process and the thinking skills used. Again, students can be encouraged to use the thinking vocabulary terms identified in Chapter 1 to describe *how* (in addition to what) they are thinking to a classmate or to the instructor.

▷▷▷▷▷Action Learning #70: Finding the Best Cluster

▷ **Rationale:** This exercise provides students with practice for the next level of thinking required for efficient, effective great nursing care. Although this task is sophisticated for beginning students, it is important for them to see what clustering as part of great nursing looks like and have an opportunity to try it.

▷ **Teaching Options:** The objective of this activity can be achieved in any setting with any data base or with a clinical patient. It may be helpful for the instructor to provide additional examples to begin to guide students in this thinking skill. Students may feel less anxious practicing this activity if they work in small groups and collaborate on the answer.

In the clinical setting, students could be asked to work with a peer to critique and offer each other suggestions. Each student would provide feedback to his or her peer regarding the effectiveness of finding the best clusters for the assigned patients for the day.

It is important for the instructor to be supportive of all efforts at this higher order thinking task and to emphasize the underlying purpose of this skill, which is to design the most effective, safe, and efficient nursing care. To communicate this support, the instructor could provide specific written feedback on written care plans, develop a special conference session to explore and practice clustering, or work with other faculty to incorporate "Finding the Best Cluster" work into other learning opportunities.

Thinking Log #12

This Thinking Log is designed to promote an understanding of the patient's unique situation. When students project themselves into the patient's role, they start to consider the feeling part of care. These feelings are a critical ingredient of caring. Stimulation of feelings also motivates students to do their best thinking. Writing helps to organize and clarify thoughts and feelings. This log could be shared in small groups or in a postconference to enhance peer collaboration.

13

Designing, Doing, and Determining Quality of Care for Actual Problems with Multiple Related Factors

Chapter 13 continues the thinking related to Betty's case as the nurse incorporates planning, implementing, and evaluating into the "big picture." This chapter begins the focus of care on actual problems with multiple related factors. Addressing multiple related factors is vital to great nursing and is often glossed over in many textbooks.

The interconnectedness of planning, implementing, and evaluating is emphasized continually to remind the student of the "big picture." The more students recognize the necessity of applying the nursing process as an integrated whole the more likely they are to achieve great nursing.

Another purpose of this chapter is to nurture the student's thinking about written care plans. Creating a care plan from scratch can produce anxiety in the beginner. This anxiety decreases thinking and learning. Providing students with existing works to critique diminishes anxiety so that thinking skills can be engaged more effectively.

Designing, Doing, and Determining Quality of Care for Actual Problems ▼ 71

▶ **Key Content Areas**

Nursing Diagnoses for Actual Problems
Multiple Related Factors for Actual Problems
Qualitative Differences in Written Plans

▶ **Teaching Objectives**

- Assist students in appreciating the interconnectedness of planning, implementing, and evaluating care based on the assessment.
- Guide students in understanding actual nursing problems and identifying multiple related factors.
- Promote skills in critiquing written care plans and modifying them to improve individualization and effectiveness of care.

Rationale and Teaching Options for Active Learning Exercises

Action Learning #71: Thoughts on Being Directive with Betty about Her Decisional Conflict

▷ **Rationale:** This exercise is designed to help students recognize that "directives" issued by nurses are not the most therapeutic. The questions are designed to specifically nurture thinking about effective ways to promote behavior change. Hopefully, students will begin to realize that great nursing care is not achieved by simply telling the patient what to do.

▷ **Teaching Options:** In the classroom or clinical setting, students could share their answers to the questions in the text. Students could also be asked what they think Betty might feel about being told she had to do something. It would be useful to ask students to share how they feel when they are told to do something they do not want to do or are not ready to do. The instructor could ask students to share some health behaviors they know they should change but haven't. Then they could explore some of the reasons why change has not occurred.

It is important to prevent the group discussion from putting other students on the spot and pressuring them to actually make the changes in behavior. One method that helps avoid that group pressure is to refocus on the purpose of the activity and remind the group that patients experience similar dilemmas when they are directed to do something. Patience and caring are essential ingredients to great nursing in these situations. This can also be a good time to discuss issues of patients' overdependence on nursing staff and how to recognize and discourage situations in which patients demonstrate unhealthy dependence.

▷▷▷▷▷▷Action Learning #72: Critique of Sue's Plan

▷ **Rationale:** This activity provides an opportunity for students to evaluate the work of an anonymous peer. As explained in the text, this process produces less anxiety than starting from scratch to develop a care plan. It also allows for application of concepts as students begin to recognize ineffective aspects of the written plan.

The Tracking Nursing Thinking (TNT) Checklist provides a structure for the student's critique. If using the TNT, the student must engage all five modes of thinking and make some beginning quality judgments about poor, good, or better quality.

▷ **Teaching Options:** In addition to the textbook care plan and discussion of the plans strengths and weaknesses, any care plan can be used for this activity in either the classroom or clinical setting. A small or large group could randomly select one care plan and evaluate its quality. It will be important to guide the group in constructive criticism techniques to diminish the anxiety of the student whose plan is selected to be reviewed. It is also helpful to have one student in the group take responsibility for verbally summarizing the suggestions and comments of the critique. Thanking the individual for sharing the plan is also a nice group gesture. During this activity, it is particularly useful for the instructor to reinforce the idea that there are many right answers or effective ways to planning care.

Another teaching option is for students to regularly "grade" each others' clinical care plans and use group discussions to share thoughts and ideas. Collaboration in care planning is extremely valuable in stimulating all modes of THINK.

Students might also be encouraged to critique and modify the TNT. They might want to add areas that would more clearly focus on the setting of their clinical activities. Or they may want to condense some areas. The more personalized the learning instruments, the better the learning.

Action Learning #73: Becoming Thelma

▷ **Rationale:** This activity builds on the learning in #72. It again asks the student to evaluate the care planning ability of an anonymous peer. This provides for repetition in applying concepts to increase retention.

The activity then provides an opportunity to fix or improve the poor plan. This approach creates less anxiety than writing one's own plan from scratch but achieves the goal of learning how to modify. It particularly nurtures the modes of INQUIRY and NEW IDEAS AND CREATIVITY.

▷ **Teaching Options:** The teaching options here are similar to those of #72. Any plan in any setting can be used as long as its focus is an actual problem with multiple related factors. The questions listed in the discussion section of the text can be helpful in guiding students to think about similarities and differences in their planning skills.

It is a good idea to encourage students to start saving all their TNTs and to keep track of their care planning strengths and weaknesses. For example, if their care plans are consistently poor or good in the area of measurability of patient objectives, this may be an indication that some learning has not occurred. Useful questions to ask might include "What does this mean?" "What is not clear?" "What do I need to change my ranking in this area?" "How can I determine improvement?"

Still another activity option is to examine existing data bases with nursing diagnoses of actual problems. The task for the individual students or the group would be to use TOTAL RECALL and INQUIRY modes of thinking to find all the related factors.

Thinking Log #13

This log encourages students to use NEW IDEAS AND CREATIVITY to develop personalized memory aids incorporating the many aspects of great care planning. The sooner the basics become second nature, the easier it will be for students to see the "big picture" and design safe, efficient, and effective care.

14

Designing, Doing, and Determining Quality of Care for High-Risk Problems

Chapter 14 is the third in this final section on examining the nurse's thinking about Betty's complex needs. The focus here is on the potential or high-risk problems. In addition to clarifying the terminology, the text examines the differences in thinking, structure, and planning between actual and high-risk problems. Recognizing these differences helps students improve their diagnostic abilities. A brief discussion of the interface of potential problems diagnosed by nurses, physicians, and other providers serves as additional clarification. As students recognize these differences, their diagnostic accuracy increases.

The remainder of the chapter describes designing, doing, and determining quality of care for Betty. Students are again given the opportunity to critique and modify a plan of care. Repetition of newly learned skills increases retention of learning.

▶ Key Content Areas

Nursing Care with High-Risk Problems
Differences between Actual and High-Risk Problems
Qualitative Differences in Written Plans

Designing, Doing, and Determining Quality of Care for High-Risk Problems

▶ **Teaching Objectives**

- Assist students in appreciating the higher levels of thinking needed to design care for high-risk problems.
- Promote skills in critique and modification of care plans.

Rationale and Teaching Options for Action Learning Exercises

Action Learning #74: What is the Risk?

▷ **Rationale:** This activity helps students apply their thinking while determining if patients are at risk for problems, what problems they may be at risk for, and what knowledge is needed to make those judgments. Students have been given an example of the thinking used for determining risk, and they can now apply that process to different situations. Repetition of the thinking with three brief situations promotes internalization of the concepts being learned.

▷ **Teaching Options:** Numerous examples from clinical situations can be substituted or added to this activity. Students could work in small groups or independently to identify patient risk factors.

An alternative project is to construct a poster or illustration of the numerous bodies of knowledge needed to identify risk factors. This illustration could include representations of all the basic sciences, the humanities, life experience, and so forth.

A third activity might be to have all students prepare two short scenarios of risk factor clusters. Students could present the scenarios to the larger group or to their clinical group. Others in the group would then describe their thinking and the knowledge used to diagnose the high-risk problems.

Action Learning #75: Becoming Thelma Again

▷ **Rationale:** This activity provides for more repetition of skills, but this time with an additional aspect of care—high-risk problems. This activity also can be used to help students recognize that repetition will allow these thinking skills to work more smoothly and efficiently.

▷ **Teaching Options:** Other plans can be substituted or added to enhance repetition and learning. It will be helpful to use situations with at least two or three risk factors as a means of encouraging students to be good health detectives.

An additional activity might include a project in which students survey nursing personnel to determine how they think about and diagnose high-risk problems. An ideal situation would be for students to interview nurses in a variety of settings—acute care, home care, well baby clinics, outpatient surgery, schools, and so forth. The added advantage of this assignment would be to identify the kinds and frequency of high-risk problems in different settings.

Thinking Log #14

This Thinking Log is designed to continue the application of care planning and thinking. This time the student is asked to particularly focus on thinking skills used. This nurtures the KNOWING HOW YOU THINK mode, which is essential for growth toward great nursing.

15

Designing, Doing, and Determining Quality of Care for Wellness Issues, Interdisciplinary Problems, and Problems for Referral

Chapter 15 concludes this section on Betty's complex problems. It addresses the aspect of nursing care that requires a good understanding of health, the role of other health care providers, and collaboration.

A brief discussion reviews the debate over wellness diagnoses and the current NANDA guidelines for use. The chapter also addresses the importance of knowing the roles and responsibilities of other disciplines to diagnose interdisciplinary problems and make effective referrals. A table is provided to help the student examine the differences and similarities among the major conclusions of assessment.

Betty's case again shows how thinking in all five modes is needed to address these major conclusions of assessment. The Action Learning exercises provide opprotunities for students to integrate these new concepts into their growing understanding of nursing care.

Designing, Doing and Determining Quality of Care for Wellness Issues

▶ Key Content Areas

Nursing Care for Wellness Diagnoses, Interdisciplinary Problems, and Problems for Referral

Differences, Similarities, and Overlap among All the Major Conclusions of Assessment

▶ Teaching Objectives

- Assist students to appreciate the thinking needed to design care for wellness diagnoses, interdisciplinary problems, and problems for referral.
- Guide students in their thinking to make accurate conclusions about wellness diagnoses, interdisciplinary problems, and problems for referral.

Rationale and Teaching Options for Action Learning Exercises

▷▷▷▷▷▷Action Learning #76: Identifying Problems for Referral

▷ **Rationale:** This activity is designed to help students recognize the influence of their knowledge base, experiences, values, and beliefs on their ability to effectively identify problems for referral. The discussion section in the text provides questions to nurture students' thinking and encourages them to justify their reasoning.

▷ **Teaching Options:** Additional scenarios could be substituted or added to the four in the exercise. As students' knowledge base grows, more sophisticated topics can be added as well.

Alternative value-laden examples could include cases of domestic violence, substance abuse, incest, religious beliefs, and so forth. The purpose of an expanded discussion on values would not be to change values as much as to increase awareness of values. Once students recognize that their values are indeed values and not necessarily universal truths, they can make more informed decisions about patient needs and patient care.

Still another activity to improve referral-making might be to interview nurses and ask what kinds of issues they usually refer and why. It might be interesting to correlate any differences with the experience level of the nurse and the setting of care. Each student could interview one nurse and compare the results to those of other students in clinical groups or in class.

Action Learning #77: Increasing Your Content Knowledge for Referring Problems

▷ **Rationale:** This activity encourages students to get first-hand knowledge of the roles and responsibilities of other providers. It creates an opportunity to talk to and discuss professional issues with other providers. Minimal structure for that interaction is provided so that a natural discovery process is used. Direct contact and understanding of the roles and responsibilities of other providers significantly increases the probablily of effective referrals. This is also an excellent start for future networking.

▷ **Teaching Options:** Instead of allowing for random selection of other providers, a list of different providers could be generated. Students could each pick a different provider for an interview to avoid excessive duplication and overwhelming one department of providers.

Another option is to have a small group of students select one specific type of provider such as physical therapists. Each student could interview a different physical therapist. The group could then compare their results and discuss differences as well as the importance of knowing specifics about agencies and individual providers. This activity would reinforce the importance of getting first-hand knowledge and not just the generalities provided in books describing physical therapy.

Still another activity might include a retroactive evaluation of referrals made by nurses over the last 6 months. Students could decide which criteria they wanted to study. Those criteria might include how the referral was made (phone, in person), how quickly the patient made contact with the other provider, and results of the referral. A discussion at the end of the assignment could focus on what the students learned about effective and efficient ways to make referrals.

Action Learning #78: Distinguishing the Category of the Conclusion of Assessment

▷ **Rationale:** This activity provides practice in using the information from Table 15.1 and applying that information to examples of patient health concerns. The better students become in accurately identifying the patient's health concerns, the better they will be at designing the most effective, safe, and efficient care. Accuracy in diagnosing is the foundation of great nursing interventions.

▷ **Teaching Options:** In a clinical setting, students could use Table 15.1 to evaluate the nurses' conclusions of assessment found in patient records. Depending on the setting, this may be a way to highlight which concerns are most likely addressed and which concerns are least likely identified. Discussion could help students hypothesize on the reasons for these trends and if the trends reflect any need to change how nursing care is delivered.

In the classroom setting, students could be divided into five groups. Each group could be asked to prepare a presentation on one of the conclusion categories. The group could provide an explanation of the category, examples from their clinical experiences, and two items for a quiz. After all the presentations are completed, the quiz items could be combined for a class quiz on the material to evaluate retention of the content.

Thinking Log #15

The primary purpose of this final Thinking Log is to encourage students to apply all the concepts they have been learning, use the TNT as a guide, and design care that considers all the major conclusions of assessment. Some patients may not have health concerns in all areas, but it is important for nursing students to consciously make that determination and not just ignore it. This final log builds on the learning with ongoing repetition to reinforce new skills.

The second purpose of this log is to emphasize the importance of keeping a Care Plan Portfolio for future reference. A portfolio provides for ongoing evaluation, close monitoring of progress, and recognition of patterns that may need improvement. It is important for students to recognize and have tangible evidence of growth in their thinking and their ability to achieve great nursing. Positive reinforcement of professional growth nurtures self-esteem and continued growth.

16

Thinking into the Future: From Linear Equation to Paradigm of Great Nursing

Chapter 16 is designed to return the student to the "big picture" after acquiring a working knowledge of the details of thinking and the nursing process. This chapter emphasizes that great nursing goes well beyond the original linear equation described in Chapter 3. That equation simply added the components of great nursing together, as if they were separate, finite entities. By this time students are beginning to see that great nursing is much more that. Students are asked to draw on their newly enhanced thinking skills and create their own personal paradigm using the components of great nursing. This personal creation nurtures both responsibility and accountability—the keys to the future of great nursing.

▶ **Key Content Areas**

    Identification of the Evolution of Thinking and Learning That Has Occurred

    Creation of a Personal Paradigm of Great Nursing

82 ▼ Thinking into the Future

▶ Teaching Objectives

- Guide students in recognizing their growth in thinking and learning.
- Assist students in using their NEW IDEAS AND CREATIVITY mode to capture their learning in a paradigm that represents their interpretation of great nursing.

Rationale and Teaching Options for Action Learning Exercises

▷▷▷▷▷▷ **Action Learning #79: Thinking Skills; #80: The Relationship between Thinking Skills and Content Knowledge; #81: The Relationship among the Nursing Process, Thinking Skills, and Content Knowledge; #82: Adding the Patient to the Diagram; #83: Incorporating the Unique You into the Diagram; #84: From Linear Equation to Paradigm**

▷ **Rationales:** These final activities are discussed as a whole because great nursing is a whole that is greater than the sum of its parts. Students are asked to build their personal paradigms by creating visual representations of the components and the relationships among the components. The outcome of this activity provides the student with ownership. This ownership enhances learning and nurtures the potential for ongoing growth.

Students are also encouraged to share their ideas and creations with classmates. This provides for continued peer collaboration and support. The suggestion is also made that they keep their paradigm and reexamine it at graduation. This puts in place the notion that this creation is not only worth saving but that it is permissible to change it as thinking and learning grow.

▷ **Teaching Options:** The authors suggest these Action Learning exercises be completed as they are described in the text. Some faculty or students may wish to add additional components to the paradigm, but it is important to keep the process of paradigm development intact. Additional components may enhance the paradigm, but the process of personally creating a paradigm and including a unique representation of the student is a powerful learning tool. This process is especially well suited for the complex learning about thinking and its role in great nursing.